Right or wrong, Chief Surgeon Haims was never slow to adopt a high moral tone and never lost a battle or confrontation. It was clearly beyond his comprehension that he could possibly lose this one.

But it was the pathologist who made the final diagnosis—a medical doctor who was impartial to doctors he served, regardless of the consequences to the individual physician or to the hospital that hired him. The patient was to be protected. No surgeon-physician was allowed to control the pathologist's diagnosis.

"You still haven't told me who you are going to tell!" queried Haims.

"Thought about it all night. I don't know," Hank Whipple answered.

The surgeon's knife was probing, trying to find the right place...."Suppose I stop? Then we'd be friends again and this could be all forgotten." A small smile lifted up the edges of Haims' thin lips, but the eyelids remained narrowed.

Whipple didn't reply....

Haims leaned forward. "I can squash you like a bug," he whispered, "like the common cockroach you are....whenever I want, Whipple! You're going to get a lesson. Watch me!"

Pathologist In Peril

Pathologist In Peril

Harry Chinchinian

Plum Tree Press
Washington

Pathologist In Peril

For information, address: Plum Tree Press
531 Silcott Road, Clarkston, WA 99403

Printing History:
First Printing 1995
Second Printing 1996

ISBN 0-9653535-2-4

Also by Harry Chinchinian
Published by Plum Tree Press:

IMMIGRANT SON
MURDER IN THE MOUNTAINS*

*Forthcoming

To Mary

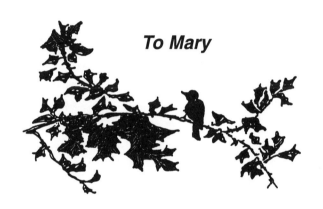

One

Hank Whipple, pathologist, sat in the hospital cafeteria and stirred his coffee as he watched John Haims, a general surgeon, approach his table.

Haims's movements were purposeful and quick, and his ceaselessly moving eyes checked everyone who passed.

"You all right now?" he stopped and drawled to an elderly man. "Check with me soon." To another he asked, "Where have you been?" It was an attentive manner that made him the busiest physician in the hospital.

Small-boned, short, tanned and hawk-faced, the earth colors of his spotless suit matched the impeccable shine on his shoes. He sat down with assurance and asked in an irritated voice, "What is it you want, Whipple?" Haims noted the orange juice that Whipple had ordered for him and drank part of the glass.

Whipple hesitated then plunged in. "Someone has been altering the diagnoses on our tissue reports. Many of the tissues you removed in surgery have been improperly re-categorized. The correct diagnosis of Uterus—no abnormal changes, has been changed to 'Multiple fibroadenomas' and often 'endometriosis' has been added. 'Appendix—normal' has been changed to 'Appendix—purulent.' In general, normal tissues have been reclassified into disease categories."

"Why approach me about this? What would I have to do with such things?" asked Haims, brushing his arm with his fingernails.

"You'd have the most to gain."

"How so?" The eyelids narrowed and angry wrinkles appeared at the edges.

"You know. Insurance companies will not pay for the removal of normal tissue in surgery without precise and lengthy documentation. They will certainly question the necessity of the operation in the first place. Also, the tissue surgery committee would begin questioning the abilities of any surgeon who—"

"These are my patients you are talking about. People who trust in my abilities and diagnoses! The tissues removed in surgery are removed by me. Only diseased, cancerous, or abnormal material is removed!" Haims's face reddened as he spoke.

Whipple looked at the windows outside the cafeteria which were streaming with pelting rain.

"Who do you think you are, interfering with my patients and my diagnoses?" continued Haims, his voice brimming with anger as he spit out words through clenched teeth.

Whipple turned away from the windows and shrugged. "My specialty takes the same number of years as yours. If anything, my academic credentials are superior. The hospital rules state that only the pathologist is allowed to diagnose, in detail, the condition and state of the tissue cut out by any surgeon. One copy of the report is sent to medical records, one copy is placed in the patient's chart, one copy goes to the attending physician and the fourth is kept on file in the laboratory permanently. The reports in medical records and in the patients' charts have all been altered."

"You needn't lecture me about who's responsible for what in a hospital!" exclaimed Haims. "I don't have time for you glorified pencil pushers and bean counters."

"Falsification of hospital documents may constitute a felony, especially if—"

"Cut the crap! Get to the point!"

Whipple looked quietly at a flustered and angry Haims. "Dr. Haims, you were involved in changing all these diagnoses. An aide reported that you were spending a lot of time talking with the medical secretary in medical records. I asked the secretary and she admitted what she was doing—under your orders."

"Whipple! Is this what I get for backing you for the job as chief of pathology!? Is this loyalty?"

"It's totally dishonest. You know it."

"Who have you told so far?" Haims asked.

"I haven't told anyone yet. It's so bizarre."

Hank Whipple looked down at the new hospital carpeting dejectedly.

The typical buzzing of voices flew around them. The new decor and carpeting had changed the drab, dreary cafeteria confines into a blend of abstract colors without warmth or identity. Sharp sounds were reduced. The corner of the hospital cafeteria where they were sitting wasn't busy but even so, their conversation was halted by many greetings from hospital workers and by the insistent loudspeaker-pager.

The silence between them was interrupted by the hospital pager: "Dr. Haims...call 332 please. Dr. Haims...332."

Haims whipped up his pager like a saber and dialed the number which was still echoing on the walls from the strident voice of the loudspeaker. He listened a moment and then decisively gave a list of orders into the phone.

Outside the hospital windows, the winter drizzle of the rain had changed to steady streams of water, rivulets cascading down the edges of the windows. He had approached Haims after lying awake all night, realizing full well how the surgeon would react to the accusation.

Haims was back in their conversation. "What makes you think I did anything wrong? It was my diagnosis! My patient! My surgery!"

"That may be," said Hank Whipple softly. "But my medical territory is the *final* anatomical diagnosis. It's what counts and it's what the hospital and other doctors depend upon for confirmation."

"Look," Haims said, leaning forward as his elbows buttressed his words. "You perceive a problem when there is no problem! It's not anything like you are trying to make out! Massaging the diagnoses just smooths the way so the hospital can get paid. You know that! Each diagnosis has a number. That's how we get paid. By numbers matching numbers. Patient care is not affected, so it's not that important."

"Why, John? You can't need the money!" Hank's eyebrows were almost knitted together.

Haims pulled the orange juice toward himself in an

irritated gesture, as if to fling the remainder somewhere. His body signals clearly predicted the barrage that was to come.

"Tell me, Whipple, since you're so high and mighty, who has the most patients at St. Mary's?"

"You do."

"You bet your sweet ass! I represent 38.5 percent of the gross income to this hospital!" Haims's voice was harshly cutting. "Would you like to tell the administrator to start charges against me?"

"No. He's in your pocket. He's salaried."

Haims smiled. "And he's going to crap when I tell him to crap! ...How about informing the president of the medical staff?"

"Havermann? Your relative."

"The chairman of tissue surgery?" continued Haims.

Whipple smiled. A joke. Haims had insisted on being the chairman of this committee for the past five years—a thankless job no one else wanted. Now, of course, it was evident why he continuously volunteered—no, insisted— on volunteering his services.

"The hospital board?" His eyes glittered with an implied threat. "Would you like to try them?"

"You've done well there, too. Half of them are your patients," Whipple guessed at the figure.

"Three-quarters," corrected Haims triumphantly and straightened up in his chair. "That's 75 percent to you! Not only patients, but personal friends! Unlike you, they know how to express their appreciation!"

Haims was defending his turf.

Right or wrong, Haims was never slow to adopt a high moral tone and never lost a battle or confrontation. It was clearly beyond his comprehension that he could possibly lose this one.

But it was the pathologist who made the final diagnosis—a medical doctor who was impartial to the doctors he served, regardless of the consequences to the individual physician or to the hospital that hired him. The patient was to be protected. No surgeon-physician was allowed to control the pathologist's diagnosis.

"You still haven't told me who are you going to tell!"

"Thought about it all night. I don't know," Hank answered.

The surgeon's knife was probing, trying to find the right place. It was clear that Haims saw him as a hospital-salaried doctor, another pencil pusher who merely sat behind a desk, and now dared to threaten his actions.

"Suppose I stop? Then we'd be friends again and this could all be forgotten." A small smile lifted up the edges of Haims's thin lips, but the eyelids remained narrowed.

Whipple didn't reply. They both were aware that Whipple's report, in the right hands, would cause an outside investigation. Haims, with his influence, could obfuscate or stonewall the exact details. At the worst, he would survive the temporary loss of his medical license but the facts would be documented and entered into the American Medical Association computer permanently and the printout of his professional life would be there for anyone to read under the Freedom of Information Act.

Haims leaned forward. "I can squash you like a bug," he whispered, "like the common cockroach you are...whenever I want, Whipple! You're going to get a lesson. Watch me!"

Shoving back his chair with a deliberate smile, Haims acted as though they had just had a friendly chat—but his footsteps left an angry tattoo in the air behind him as he walked out.

Hank stood up and held the coffee to his lips. Although the cup was still full, the liquid was cold. As he tasted it, he felt an intestinal churning.

"Hank," said a voice in his ear. "You look like hell. Why don't you stop drinking?"

It was Tom Deakis, obstetrician, and recently Hank's charge under the PRN—the Physician's Recovery Network—which handled physicians with chemical dependencies.

"Drinking?" Hank was slow to see the humor. Tom was forced to urinate under observation, without forewarning, and submit the sample to Hank for alcohol analysis. Drinking was Tom's problem. No one was officially allowed to know Tom was under surveillance, including the medical staff. But there were no secrets, even in the largest of hospitals.

"Sure. Let me blow my breath on Haims and he'll dissolve from shock, if nothing else—like all teetotalers! You look like you were having trouble," said Deakis curiously.

"Always something, isn't there." Hank Whipple, with effort, managed to summon a weak grin as he headed back to the laboratory.

What was going to happen now?

His father-in-law, the financier, would have seen the irony in his situation. Approving of his choice in medicine, he often wondered aloud at Hank's choice of specialty.

"I'm told only people who want to hide go into laboratories," he said. "When you can't get along with anybody, there's the last refuge. Into the laboratory. Hide in research. A trade-off for security."

Security?

After a rotating internship where he sampled all of the departments of medicine, Hank had decided the laboratory was far more challenging. It meant a salaried position—not something his father-in-law really approved of, but accepted. Entrepreneurs had little patience with salaried people. His father-in-law risked and gained but had decided Hank was a no-risk, no-gain type.

Hank smiled ruefully. His father-in-law had no concept of his work and the risks, much less his character.

He was a salaried physician with no independent income. His wife Corky would back him, but at age forty-five and with three children, it would be difficult to pick up and move.

Would he be able to keep his job? Or would Haims smear him?

Two

Hank's microscope lay open. One of his partners must have been using it. A questionable blood smear was left by the technologist for interpretation by a pathologist. He glanced at the blood count and who had performed it. Satisfied that it was performed in their own laboratory, he relaxed as he focused down on the individual cells which were stained purple, blue and red with Wright's Stain.

"Atypical cells" was written on the report. "Rule out lymphocytic leukemia."

Marilyn Meagen, the hematology supervisor, enjoyed misleading him. Leukemia could have a high or low white blood cell count but this was a smear of infectious mononucleosis. The large transformed lymphocytes had bland nuclei and a ballerina-skirt type of cytoplasm. A high white blood count and almost all lymphocytes, certainly, but not leukemia.

He walked out into the hematology area and said, "Serious case of pharngitis?"

Meagen smiled but did not pause in her work, since blood counts were a priority in the early morning.

"Heterophile positive," she called over her shoulder.

Heterophile was a test for Infectious Mononucleosis—a benign disease that mimicked leukemia.

"Positive heterophiles occur in leukemia, too. A report is probably somewhere in the literature," he admonished, returning the smile to her back now.

"Anything can be reported in the literature," she replied without turning around. "Anything!" she emphasized, still not looking up but expertly adjusting the microscope with a minimal of motion.

The surgeon Sam Sager walked in. He looked and acted like a big gray-headed bear, about two hundred fifty pounds and five-ten.

"Hi, everybody! Give me some cheerful news for a change! Does Jonathan Peterson have leukemia? Say no! Please!"

"No!" Hank and Marilyn replied together.

Sam looked almost ready to cry with relief as he waved his large hands in the air. "Is that right? With that huge white count and all those ecchymoses? You have made me very happy! He's my golfing buddy—the only one I can beat. You have no idea how important it is to me! This is wonderful! I love you laboratory people!" said Sam, genuinely pleased. Well, thought Hank, once in a while the laboratory can provide good news, even when it appears clinically serious.

Sam Sager left, but shortly, Hank knew, they would receive a bouquet of flowers and a box of candy. It was a pleasure working for some of the doctors.

Nervous movements everywhere. Blood sugars, blood-clotting tests, bilirubins—all chemical elements of the human body were being analyzed by the computerized medical instrumentation and continuously checked for accuracy by the internal and external quality controls. Then a button was pressed by the medical technologist and the blood-test values sped electronically to the doctor and to the medical or surgical floors.

Excessively high or low values, that is, life-threatening increases or decreases of chemicals in the bloodstream, were phoned immediately to the physician. These were called panic values. Every laboratory was required to post them and notify the doctors as soon as the analysis was completed.

That's what made the laboratory the most important part of the hospital. Patients were quickly treated for their aliments based on lab analyses.

The laboratory was a comfort, Hank thought, as he returned to his room. It was like being on a ship, a solid, well-run ship, which was handled by a capable and skillful crew. Or was he simply taking refuge? Hiding behind books and research—just as his father-in-law said? Whatever. It was something he didn't think much about, until now.

He was proud of his work and his crew. *His* crew?

No. Not really. They were hospital employees, as were his three colleagues, none of whom would support any type of confrontation with any doctor or administrator.

He took a deep breath and stretched before he began reviewing the difficult or abnormal Pap smears screened by the cytologist.

His changed relationship with Haims would not go unnoticed.

Countless small pranks relieved the tedium in surgery. The sudden lack of humor between Haims and Whipple would be immediately noticed. The hospital was large, but not large enough to escape nuances between personalities. The surgical department was fine-tuned to everything affecting the operations. Surgeons, assistants and nurses were shuffled according to ability as well as personality.

Avoiding confrontations was paramount for a smooth work-flow in any hospital. He had acquired a powerful enemy, an enemy that was like a huge, smoldering fire below the waterline in a ship, poorly contained by its wooden structure. The acrid smoke would lift up through the air ducts and stairways, seep through the planks and sleeping quarters, and would eventually spread to the deck with its ugly black and red teeth.

His comfortable refuge—surrounded as he was by scholarly books and erudite lecture notes, slides and tapes— was, at best, temporary and vulnerable.

How soon the attack?

Three

The expected smoke and flames came from below the bow of the ship in the form of a summons from the administrator of the hospital the next morning.

It was a bland telephone request asking Hank to meet with him, at his convenience, in his office, but that afternoon.

Administration had multiple offices on the lobby floor. Because it was the lobby, the carpeting was thick and the room was surrounded by large and small plants. The auxiliary shop had cut flowers displayed outside and also on the reception desk. The volunteers at the information desk smiled at him as they smiled at everyone who walked by.

The administrator's door was open and easily seen from his secretary's office. His door was never closed.

The administrator's desk was clear except for neatly piled papers in one corner. It could have been any office anywhere, except for the mementos and award plaques on the north wall. Only then did you realize how impressive were the achievements of the inhabitant.

Tim Hawkes, the administrator, was black—as was his wife. They were overachievers, originating from New York, compulsive about education to the point of earning several master's degrees in unrelated fields. Tim had a master's in botany and also in business administration. A puzzling combination. His wife taught nursing and was a CPA. An equally puzzling combination. Together, as personalities, they were formidable.

Wisely, both had said they kept their job options open for the simple reason that hospital administrators were politically vulnerable. Multiple fund-raising campaigns were an on-going state of affairs and as a result, everyone who contributed to the hospital felt free to criticize hospital management. If that weren't enough, critics included the St. Mary's nuns in Minneapolis who actually owned the hospital, the board of directors, the local newspaper, patients and their relatives, the medical staff and the hospital staff.

Tim walked the thin wire agilely and was never known to show anger—especially over racial or personal slights. Bigots grudgingly gave them good marks for community service.

"You're looking thin, Hank," said Tim Hawkes.

Hank sat down and looked at the mementos and award plaques carefully placed around Tim's desk.

"No. I stay the same," said Hank. "I see you've added another award."

A standing joke between them. Awards impressed Tim's bosses—the nuns in Minneapolis—so he displayed them when necessary on their visits and took them down when they left. He had forgotten to take down the last group of awards.

Tim was solemn. "How are things going?"

"You're about to tell me and I don't think it's going to be good." Hank sat prepared.

Tim flushed slightly and his hands folded and refolded, reflecting the agitation in his mind.

On a professional level, Hank felt he knew him as well as anyone. Sober, traditional, Tim was careful to follow the orthodox establishment outlook.

"Doctor, as you know, the hospital is always on a budget..." He looked at Hank for a reaction.

The hospital had just finished dunning the medical staff for the latest building program, "suggesting" a $5,000 donation from each member. Hospitals always lost money but managed, one way or another, to keep on building bigger and bigger structures.

When Hank smiled, Tim realized poor-mouthing was the wrong opening, gave a self-deprecating laugh, and bought time to switch his gambit by carefully removing a cigarette from the pack and lighting it deliberately and slowly. Curious it was to Hank that Tim adamantly refused to give up smoking in spite of the multitude of critics.

Tim took the sledgehammer approach. "We need to save money," he said abruptly. "Dr. Schmidt is willing to run the lab as director. You are going to be asked to stay on as staff pathologist."

"Salary?"

"$60,000."

"Half," Hank said.

Tim looked embarrassed and shuffled some papers.

Hank stretched out his legs and exhaled slowly as he said, "Offering half-salary is the same as asking someone to leave, of course. It's the easy way of getting rid of a problem worker. How about Schmidt's salary?"

"Well…" Tim looked down at the papers on his desk. "About $80,000…for now."

"Negotiable?"

"Not…for…with you," he finished lamely.

"Pressure from Haims, Tim?" Hank asked.

Tim didn't answer and started to reach for his lighter to light the cigarette which was already lit in his hand.

A primary law in jungle fighting is to always stay under cover and never become a target. If someone else wants to become a target, it's his business. For whatever reason, Hank had made himself a target. The reason was inconsequential. A target was a target and got blown away.

A smart survivor had options of either getting out of the way of the target, eliminating the target, eliminating the threat or getting out of the battle area. It was easiest eliminating the target: Hank.

Tim was only doing his job. People posing as threats were dispensable. The smooth flow of hospital operations must never be interrupted for one person. Team players were required. When you weren't a member of the team, you were swept out, no matter the reason.

They both looked at each other, fully understanding what was transpiring and yet not giving voice to their thoughts.

Hank shook his head. "Do I have time to think it over?"

The unexpected surrender startled Tim. Relief flooded over his face. "Oh, take your time. There's no hurry. Dr. Schmidt will begin tomorrow, unless…"

The word *unless*, he left hanging. It meant, "Are you going to make trouble?"

Would it do any good to explain what he had found? That his diagnoses were changed? Falsified? When was a diagnosis falsified and when was it *massaged*, as Haims put it?

At the last hospital staff meeting, doctors were admonished that revenue had decreased because diagnoses were not listed properly, so payment was not obtained. Upgrading medical and surgical diagnoses so the insurance coverage would be more was another topic. Too many doctors were placing the minimal amount of information in the discharge notes, often ignoring the multiple diseases that had been treated while the patient was in the hospital. A laundry list of all that was possible for increased revenue from the third-party payers, as Medicare and the insurance companies were termed, was handed out.

Tim cleared his throat. "I don't like doing this, Hank. It certainly isn't my idea. Let's continue being friends."

Hank got up to leave and Tim insisted on shaking hands.

Back at the office, Hank's eyes began to hurt and he rubbed them, realizing he had been up much of the night. Indecision was always wearing. He had wanted to avoid directly approaching Haims and yet knew it had to be done. Should he have gone to someone else and presented the falsification of records? Then his conscience would have been cleared, even if nothing were done and things had gone on being the same. But he knew nothing would have changed.

Deep-six it. Ignore it. Don't get involved. That's what most people did. It had nothing to do with the job description and could only lead to trouble. Take no chances and you won't get hit. It's a good living, why make waves? He knew those answers. His colleagues were part of the norm. The consequences he had avoided considering completely.

Performing diagnostic work would be a poor idea right now. His mind had to be uncluttered and his eyes were demanding rest from lack of sleep. He signed out to his colleagues, much to the surprise of the lab secretary.

Corky had gone to the Roundup Grounds to feed and exercise the horses. It was a holiday and the children were out of school. The house was quiet.

Hank was grateful just to crawl into bed and sleep.

Four

Sleep is supposed to bank the fires of the mind but sometimes it rekindles the flames from memories hidden in the odd neuron circuits of the brain.

Hank's sleep was broken with a recurrent dream.

The dream followed the same pattern: it was final exam day and Hank was about to take the last exam in an important course in order to graduate. The questions were handed out and as Hank read them, he realized none of the questions was familiar. Hank didn't know a single answer. Worse yet, he couldn't remember ever taking the course or attending class. Somehow, he also knew that if he failed this course, he would flunk out of school completely.

He watched all of his classmates writing answers to the exam questions vigorously and without hesitation. He was the only one in the room who was not writing.

Panic seized him and kept increasing more and more until he finally woke up in a sweat, his heart beating rapidly, his body shaking. For several minutes he remained convinced the event was true and that he had indeed failed.

He slowly regained his senses and began to eliminate the conviction and realized it was a just a dream, the same dream that returned, over and over.

He poured himself a cup of coffee and found a piece of apple pie. Things felt better.

It was a relief to know the consequences of his actions in confronting Haims, regardless. Indecision or waiting for bad news was always the worst part.

He had slept a few hours. It was the usual day and time for going to the Roundup Grounds—a pleasant, relaxed place filled with ranchers, cowboys and riders.

Real people. One of the major benefits of living and working in the town of Red Wolf. Everything was but ten minutes away, driving time. Relief from the hospital atmosphere was quick and complete.

He drove down to the Grounds which was located along the Clearwater River and parked next to the horse stalls. In the distance he could see Corky and the children.

Lou Gavins, the grounds manager, had acquired another stray animal. Primarily a horseman, Gavins liked all animals, bar none. People brought injured animals to him like they did to a veterinarian—this time, an injured doe. As with the others, he'd nurse it back to health and let it go.

Lou had retired from ranching but quickly found he still had to be around animals in order to enjoy life. He was a God-send to the Rodeo Board, since his qualifications were exactly what was needed for a groundskeeper. Perpetually cheerful, tall, thin to the point of emaciation, Lou always wore a large straw hat, even in the winter.

Watching Lou was Cliff Evers, a twenty-six-year-old wrangler, sitting on a bale of hay. Wordlessly, he shifted over for Hank but hardly nodded to Hank's greeting. Why? Hank could only guess.

Cowboys were a different breed. They could discuss the most intimate details about breeding animals and their sexual activities but became embarrassed about their own human needs and wants. Cliff had a serious problem: atrophied testicles, a result of a post-surgical abscess complication. Haims had performed the surgery. Was he getting proper hormone replacement therapy? Who was his doctor now? Hank didn't know. Surgeons like Haims lost interest in patients after the surgery was finished. The patients were afterward referred—probably to Dr. Span, Haims's shadow and lackey, who was in family practice.

He resolved to talk to Cliff about his condition the next time he saw him in the lab. Right then, Cliff didn't appear receptive and it would be easier on territory other than on the Roundup Grounds.

They both quietly watched Lou, who was talking softly and moving slowly in the stall with his charge. The doe was timid and frightened. It wouldn't eat and stayed as far away as it could in the corner. Eventually, Lou got it to eat a little leafy alfalfa, although nervously. It was a start. Within a few days, Lou would have it not only eating out of his hand, but on the road to health. Then, like the other animals, it would follow him around, bonded like a puppy dog. He had a real knack with animals. Taking time was an essential part, but the willingness to take the time was his strong point.

Corky was busy riding in the far arena, the children flying behind her. He could see her bobbing up and down at the extended trot and hear the loud, encouraging cries of their three children, trying to keep up with her horse.

He shouted into a herd and Crum, his gelding, ran up from the pasture, paused, smelled him and then placed his head on Hank's chest and pushed. It was his way of saying, "Let's move out."

After brushing him down and feeding him a cup of oats, Hank saddled him. This time, they'd ride into the back hills. Crum needed a change out of the arena and Hank needed the exercise.

No use telling Corky about the problems he had at the laboratory. Problems of his own devising could wait.

The hills were beautiful. The winter sun shone brightly and the brown sagebrush spotted the earth like chocolate bits on a cookie. A few birds flew up and Crum's eyes flickered at them.

When the ride was finished, man and horse were sweating and relaxed. After brushing Crum down, Hank left the area. A little over an hour had elapsed.

On the drive back, he wondered how soon the word would be out that he was no longer the director. Hospitals, like all institutions, were quick to communicate newsworthy items.

• • •

The moment he entered the lab, he realized everyone knew. Marilyn Meagen, the hematology supervisor with whom Hank had bandied words for years, didn't come in or greet him as usual. The secretaries and techs all kept their eyes busily down on their work and acted excessively preoccupied and quiet. Dead quiet—except for the hum of the medical instruments and occasional raucous printer— so that the ringing of the telephones jarred the heavy atmosphere.

The exception was his chief tech, who walked by and tried to greet him normally, but the greeting was overly warm. The chief tech turned and shuffled back to his office, studiously looking down on the paper he was carrying.

The laboratorians were sympathetic, but the situation was not of their making. Committing themselves would be aligning oneself politically and that would be courting disaster for themselves. Tomorrow, they would be themselves again and ask curious questions; today, seeing their boss reduced in authority reminded them of their own job vulnerability.

There were four pathologists working at St. Mary's. Alex Lewis, Edward Wilkins, Stan Schmidt and Hank. Duties were rotated every three months. One doctor rotated around the different outlying small hospitals and handled their labs. Two pathologists worked in surgical pathology, performing frozen sections at surgery and diagnosing excised abnormal tissues removed from the body. One pathologist worked in clinical pathology, interpreting all abnormal values of blood analyses and was responsible for discussing the findings with the clinicians. But their duties overlapped and whoever was available performed the work.

Right now, Alex was rotating; Edward was handling the surgical anatomic tissue analysis in the afternoon; Stan Schmidt and Hank were involved in surgical anatomic work in the morning and also covered blood chemistries and autopsies.

"Important meeting half an hour before the three-thirty review of malignancy diagnoses—my room!" Whipple spoke to each pathologist, interrupting their work. None seemed surprised.

While waiting, Whipple stared at the window which viewed the sidewalk. How would he present his blowup with Haims? None were beholden to him—they had been hired by St. Mary's. Their personalities did not blend easily. Pathology attracted introverted, scholarly types exemplified by Alex. They did their diagnostic work, did it exceptionally well and accurately, and after that, it was up to the attending physician to treat the patient.

The most difficult part was the diagnosis—the easiest part, the treatment. "Give me the correct diagnosis and I'll trust an intelligent person to look up most treatments in the PDR—*Physician's Desk Reference*," said one of their teachers in their medical school. Another was fond of saying, "Let me talk to the patient and get a history—the physical exam I will trust to a second-year medical student." Not quite true, of course, but enough of the truth for most ailments.

But still, it was the diagnosis that counted and that's what pathologists did—make the diagnoses.

Stan Schmidt came in early, glancing around as though noting what changes he would be making in the room. He sat down heavily, twisted his corpulent body in the chair and glowered at nothing in particular. His black mustache quivered. Alex and Ed came in shortly after.

Whipple began. "For several weeks, I've been tracing discrepancies in my diagnoses. Normal tissue removal has been recategorized on the patients' charts and in the record room by someone who is quite knowledgeable about medical terms. A secretary in medical records had been recruited. I confronted Dr. Haims about it—in less than a diplomatic manner—since they seemed to involve his surgical specimens.

"Dr. Haims did not confess or deny the connection. He did tell me to mind my own business or he would teach me a lesson in the form of 'squashing a cockroach.'"

Only Alex stirred and made a grunting noise. The others sat still and made no comment. It was worse than Whipple thought. There was no empathy—whatsoever.

He continued, reluctantly. "I would have you believe that there is a direct relationship with my demotion from director of this laboratory and the confrontation."

Legs and eyes shifted uneasily. Again, only Alex showed any emotion and that was an incoherent grunting sound.

"Is that it?" Stan Schmidt asked. "Of course, you're only presenting your side of the conversation."

"Yes, but the facts can be substantiated. Suggestions? Plan of action?" Whipple looked for a reaction. Silence. Salaried employees.

"To get along, you go along—otherwise, you get out!" Schmidt looked at the other pathologists belligerently.

No one spoke except Alex. "Ah. The wisdom of practicality has been rendered in an aphorism," he muttered sardonically.

"I've been appointed director," said Schmidt softly. "Any problem with my appointment?" He looked directly at Alex.

Alex closed his eyes briefly and gazed at the wall.

Ed yawned. "I've got work to do. Any turf fighting is your problem, not mine."

Schmidt turned and looked at Whipple. "That's it then. Sometimes when people get older, they can't bend. Things have to be their way or not at all."

They got up and left. If Hank had expected something, he would have been disappointed. Still, their lack of response left him numb.

• • •

Alex was the last to leave. He leaned over Hank's desk and whispered, "Haims has it in for others on the staff, you know. He's chased away more than a half-dozen surgeons who managed to apply and get on our staff. Only Sam Sager has managed to hold on—and he hasn't spoken to Haims in years!"

"I wasn't aware of that! Sam gets along with everyone and is so well-liked! Today he complimented us, as usual."

"Well…maybe going to the same church and having gone to the same school as Haims exempts him from a real attack. It's going to be a tough haul for you from here on…is it going to be worth it?" Alex looked at him searchingly, as though to divine his inner resolve.

"I think so. We've been very happy here."

"Well." Alex paused in thought. "Eventually, these angry types self-destruct. The question is not whether but how long."

"Thanks for the encouragement, Alex," said Hank, surprised.

Alex had hardly left when Schmidt came in with his personal possessions—pictures for the wall, a few books and his microscope in a carrying case.

"No use waiting," he said. He placed a chain of command map on the door, detailing who were in the upper and lower echelons of authority and posted several copies throughout the laboratory. Obviously, it was something he had typed up during the night.

Hank watched him bustle around the room and reflected that Schmidt was acceptable to the medical staff as director. More so than he was. For five years now, Schmidt had extended himself to be likable to the point of obsequiousness. He endeared himself in sports by losing a sufficient number of times to the right people and flattered them about their work and their medical abilities. His memory was unfailingly prodigious about their personal lives—including the names of their wives and children. Whipple could remember but a few dozen.

Schmidt's remark on people getting older left a significant piranha bite—or was it a deep, slashing wound? As in the sea, the more the victim bled, the weaker he became and the more aggressively assault wounds were inflicted by others.

Perhaps he was too old and unbending. Why be squeamish about something someone else was doing as long as it wasn't his personal business?

No. It was irresponsible to allow a coverup. A tacit sanctioning of lies demeaned the office of the laboratory director as well as his abilities as a physician.

Well, it was over. The half-salary offer was meant to be enough of an affront to make him quit. With the loss of the money was the power and prestige of the directorship. Staying on as a staff pathologist would demean his authority and influence. People would wonder about the reason and Schmidt would be predictable with innuendoes which would be untraceable. Hank could hear the whispers now: "There was a problem with his diagnoses..."

It was 3:30 P.M. He got up to join the other pathologists in reviewing the day's diagnoses of malignancies on surgical tissues and blood smears.

Five

The next morning, a letter was placed on his desk from an ad hoc committee, organized two years ago as quality assurance, an offshoot from John Haims's tissue-surgery committee.

His heart sank at what he read—there were a list of allegations and he was ordered to appear before the committee and explain certain *serious discrepancies* in pathological diagnoses at 10 A.M. the next day, Thursday.

Like all hospital committees, it was legally protected for any remarks they cared to make, slanderous or otherwise, as long as it could be shown that the remarks were made in good faith. Ostensibly it's purpose was, as the name sounded, to assure quality patient care. In reality, it had the authority to harass any doctor by subjecting him or her to such continuous reviews of their work that the practice of medicine became unbearable.

Dr. Fuller Span, Haims's protege, was chairman.

Serious discrepancies could mean anything. It was a catch basin for innumerable things. Usually, it meant the pathologist brought up his slides and reports to confirm the error a practitioner had made. Generally, it had to do with the removal of normal tissue. Other times, the surgeon was chastised for incompletely excising a tumor.

The tables were turned. Instead of confirming a problem through the pathologist, the pathologist himself was to be reviewed. If this was the case, why hadn't they given him a list of the problem diagnoses so he could review the slides and tissues? He tried to phone Dr. Span but could not reach him.

Thursday came quickly enough.

He went to the Conference Room and found Tom Deakis, the obstetrician, waiting outside the doors. So Tom had been summoned as well.

Tom Deakis was a general practitioner who, in delivering babies, had lost the last two due to his carelessness in recognizing the mothers had gestational diabetes. For eight years, he had a partner, Roger Walters, who was adept and kindly, protecting Tom and helping him in surgery whenever anything sticky came up. Roger died suddenly of a coronary and a few months later, Tom's wife died from a thrombo-embolus. With his two main supports gone, Tom came to realize quickly how completely he had depended on both of them.

His partner's patients left for other physicians. As more and more doctors opened up practices in town, his patient load went down. To occupy himself when alone, which was more and more often, he began to drink.

Slowly, almost imperceptibly, he began increasing the volume of alcohol and began to look forward to the late afternoons. It was only a small step further for him to hide a bottle in the desk drawer and begin drinking a little earlier. A little earlier became even earlier, until he had to begin the day with a shot.

On his hangover days, he made schedule changes and when the problem became more overt, denial of any loss of skill set in. What patients he had managed to retain, he began to lose, and this additional depressing factor combined with more spare time, inserted him into a vicious cycle of drinking, hangovers and depression.

It was common hospital gossip that the loss of the last two births he delivered was due to negligence and that something had to be done. This was probably why Tom was being reviewed.

Tom Deakis sat quietly outside the meeting room. His usual open-necked, colored sport shirt had been replaced by a white dress shirt and tie. His suit was well-pressed and his shoes were shined. Tom usually wore white shoes spattered with blood. This was a harmless affectation on Tom's part, a rather amusing leftover from internship days when you were proud to be doing real work instead of reading and passing exams. Blood-spattered shoes had a shock effect, Tom insisted, in that it helped collect the baby delivery bills. Parents and relatives remembered the blood-spattered shoes and the surgical gown.

Now, Tom was slung over in his chair with his chin resting on the top of another chair as though he knew what was coming; over the years, he had been on numerous committees himself, and had seen many doctors lose their privileges for just cause.

As soon as Tom saw Hank, he sat up and began explaining about the delivery problems with the two babies—unburdening himself to a fellow physician who would be uncritical and sympathetic.

"You know, Hank, not everyone agrees on what exactly constitutes diabetes in a pregnant woman."

"True. There are at least two sets of criteria in the three-hour glucose tolerance tests," said Hank.

"You know, many tests are abnormal in a pregnant woman. How excited should I become over every low or high value? I don't know."

"It's difficult to follow up on every abnormal test, but today they're fairly vigorous in identifying maternal risk factors that they didn't consider a few years ago," Hank observed.

Tom looked glum. "So many new tests to learn and consider."

They were interrupted by Dr. Fuller Span, who opened the door and ran his fingers through the thin, long hairs on his balding head.

"Come in, Whipple," he said with a scowl.

The atmosphere in the room was glacial. Besides Span, four other doctors were in the room: Steve Short, a urologist; Doug Adventi, an internist; Dick Petersman, an internist known for his irritability, and a newly minted family practitioner whose name escaped him.

Whipple felt unarmed. None were his close friends. Peevish Petersman took delight in cutting up other doctors.

Span began to read a list of diagnoses that had been labeled questionable or wrong.

"These cases of Whipple's form a pattern." he said, not looking at Hank. "It cannot be ignored any longer. The incompetence shown was, for some reason, unnoticed in the past but cannot be tolerated anymore. We owe it to our patients."

Hank sat there looking dumb, staring at Dr. Span, until he realized his mouth was open. He closed it.

Accepting the list of cases, Hank began to read them while a few of the committee members made impatient, exasperated sounds at his slowness.

"I don't recall these cases offhand," Hank protested. "We make over 6,000 tissue diagnoses a year. Terminology changes. In the past year, much has changed. A diagnosis may be perfectly acceptable for a certain time period but not in the present one. I see some diagnoses in gray areas in which disagreement is common. They are, for the most part, difficult lesions and I gave my opinion."

"We thought you would say that and checked with other pathologists who disagree and say your interpretations border on the criminal."

Hank ignored him and began reading more carefully. Pap smears he had diagnosed as moderate dysplasia showed no lesion upon tissue biopsies. There were five cases. The follow-ups were single biopsies by the surgeons and were notoriously insufficient for a survey of an entire cervix. The pathologists had gone over and over this problem of inadequate biopsies, but to no avail. Gynecologists had been taught in their culposcopy workshops that all lesions could be seen. It wasn't true. Culposcopy was basically using a magnifying lens to view the surface of the cervix. The cervix was not a smooth highway, but a compact range of mountains, where tumors could hide in the nooks, crannies and valleys.

Flipping the page, Hank observed differences between what he had diagnosed and what was subsequently found. They involved lymphomas—cancer of the lymph glands.

"Look," Hank said, "diagnoses involving lymphomas are universally accepted as being difficult in subclassification. Experts disagree. These have been dredged up from years past—when antibody tests were not available. I don't see where patient care was compromised. Nothing was called benign when it was malignant and nothing was diagnosed as malignant that was subsequently benign!"

"How about that cancerous breast tumor you missed, then? The cystosarcoma phylloides case? You called it a fibroadenoma!" Span glowered.

"It is classified under the general category of fibroadenomas. It is a benign tumor—"

"It's a *sarcoma*! Sarcoma means cancer!" Span interrupted. "Or are you going to deny that the word sarcoma means cancer?"

"The term cystosarcoma is a misnomer...was a misnomer, even one hundred fifty years ago when the tumor was first described and named. Very few of these are cancerous. I've never seen a cancerous one, except as an unknown in the workshops. Cystosarcomas are rare tumors—we'll see probably one a year."

"You still didn't call it correctly, did you? Or are you going to try to lie about it?"

"No. It's often difficult, sometimes impossible, to tell the difference between a giant fibroadenoma, cellular fibroadenoma, adenofibroma, atypical fibroadenoma and cystosarcoma phylloides. The World Health Organization has tried to clear up the misleading language. They're all in the same family and it's a judgment call."

Span triumphantly looked at the other members. "We anticipated you would deny you made a wrong diagnosis and try to sneak around an honest explanation. Your attitude confirms our decision. Your dishonesty forces us to take immediate steps or jeopardize the lives of our patients and the hospital's reputation. Your actions border on the criminal."

A vision of John Haims presented itself and stood over

Span. The narrow eyes and thin mouth hissed, "Squash you like a bug…cockroach…" And that's what was happening; Hank was being penciled out.

"At least I should have copies of any questioned diagnoses," Hank heard himself saying.

"Copies of these erroneous diagnoses and others have been sent to you by registered mail." Span stared at him emotionlessly. "The least you should have done, when you didn't know the right diagnosis, was to sent the slides away for a consultant's opinion."

Hostile thrust after hostile thrust.

Span was trying to get him to explode. Hank glanced at the faces around the table for any reaction. It was clear what Span was trying to do. These colleagues—fellow physicians who had been grateful for his expert advice—were now acting like his unresponsive fellow pathologists. They could have been strangers now. Did they really believe him guilty? A menace to their patients?

"This report goes to the executive committee?" Hank heard himself ask. The executive committee ruled on further action regarding staff privileges.

"Of course," replied Span coldly. "Until the review and final decision, the other three pathologists have been asked to check and verify each and every diagnosis and interpretation you perform."

"Each and every." He could feel an ironic smile light on his face. His colleagues would be checking his work as if he were a medical student.

"That's all, Doctor. You may go."

Hank walked out the door and avoided looking at Tom Deakis. This type of committee was out for blood and would make short work of Tom's mistakes.

Hank was, for all practical purposes, out of a job, unless

he complied with their recommendation. Having others review his work was even more demeaning and meant to be so. It was like the proposal of half-salary—it said very clearly, "Leave. We don't want you around."

On his way home for lunch, his beeper went off. The telephone number was listed. He rang it. It was Tom, his voice shaking but wanting to communicate with someone who would listen and perhaps understand.

Tom's first words were of commiseration—for Hank.

"Nice of you to take the time and trouble, Tom."

"Naw! You never did anything wrong that I can remember. On the contrary, you were a great help lots of times."

"Appreciate your saying that."

"How bad was it?" asked Tom.

It was no use keeping it a secret, Hank thought. "As bad as it could be. How about you?"

"They told me no more deliveries without a consultant with me for one year."

Hank tried to keep the surprise from his voice. That was hardly a slap on the wrist. "Is that what you are going to do?" he managed to ask.

"Haven't decided. I'm sixty-eight years old now. Malpractice insurance keeps going up. Insurance companies keep paying less and hassling more. I don't know why I keep on, but I love medicine, you know." Tom's voice slipped lower to almost a mumble. "I have some personal problems that need to be worked out...by the way...Sam Sager, the general surgeon, was also there. The committee was investigating him. What has he done?

"No idea," said Hank, trying to keep his voice noncommittal. Because he was having trouble, he wasn't going to revel in the problems of others. Yet it was a shock that Haims's alter ego was reprimanding Sam Sager—one of the four general surgeons. Had Sager crossed Haims once too often? Alex had mentioned they hadn't spoken to each other for years. He hoped the quality assurance committee didn't slash at Sam's surgical work too inappropriately.

Hank listened as Tom talked on about the unusual cases he had worked on—all which Tom felt he had resolved brilliantly. Most of them were six or seven years back; they were hazy in Hank's memory, but they were all fresh and detailed in Tom's mind. Those were the pleasant days when his wife was alive and his partner shouldered more of the burden than Tom could allow himself to believe.

Hank wondered if he was doing the same thing? Was his own work marginal and was he, too, avoiding acknowledging the importance of his own partners? First-time malignant diagnoses were reviewed daily at three-thirty in conference and even more often, there were impromptu sessions—but the decision was ultimately his on how to sign out the report. Was the committee right?

That night, after the children had settled in bed, Hank stayed up and tried to read, but his mind kept wandering. Corky had fallen asleep on top of the bed, her book still open. The house was quiet.

Hank decided to take a walk along the river road. It was a cool, slightly windy night. The ponds were partially frozen with splashes of white, brown and gray. Deep in his thoughts, he realized how much time had gone by only when he looked at his watch. It was after 1 A.M.

He returned home, he failed to awaken a sleepy Corky, who still lay on top of the bed. He rolled her one way to open the covers and rolled her back into bed, ignoring her protests.

Six

The telephone woke him from a deep sleep. It rang and rang like a fire alarm. Hank always felt surprised when the rings communicated a message themselves—the soft rings for a social conversation were quite different that the harsh, insistent rings for bad things. These rings had the harsh sound.

"Dr. Whipple?" It was three o'clock in the morning.

He recognized the voice of the police chief, Bill Enzer. Yep! It was a bad one, all right.

"Lo, Chief. What's up?"

"Difficult case we need you to check out. Suicide versus murder."

"Who?"

"Dr. Haims."

"Which patient?"

"No. Haims himself. He's dead."

"What?" Hank groped in surprise for words. "Haims is dead?"

"Right. Dr. Haims. We're at his home now and we'll need a post. Gunshot wound. Can you come out?"

"Sure," Hank replied slowly, "I'll be out as soon as I get my equipment."

The telephone had woken Corky. "I'll never understand why they can't wait until morning to call you for autopsies! A dead person isn't going anywhere!"

She sleepily got up and began making coffee. "Did I hear right? Dr. Haims is dead?"

"Yes. Gunshot wound."

"Oh!" Corky's eyes widened as she comprehended what he said.

Hank dressed and drove to the morgue for his equipment.

• • •

When he arrived at the Haims's home about fifteen minutes later, Stan Schmidt was already there.

"What brings you here?" Hank asked him with surprise.

"Switchboard notified me," he said. "The committee said I was to check out all your cases. I'm sure they meant forensic autopsies as well."

Hank looked at Schmidt and felt the anger rising. Forensics had nothing to do with the hospital. Schmidt had spoken without modulating his voice, so that everyone could hear their conversation.

"Chief," Hank said. "Officially, this will have to be Dr. Schmidt's case.

Chief Enzer had heard the conversation. He shrugged his shoulders. One pathologist was as good as another, as far as his work was concerned. He simply needed someone to help document the death. From there, he would work out whether it was natural, suicide or homicide.

The police photographers finished their work. The crime lab was coming down from Coeur d'Alene to do the more detailed work in the room.

Haims was in a leather winged-back chair and next to it was a movable elbow-type floor lamp, a Stiffel, with a tray. A partially opened book lay on the tray of the lamp. Hank curiously read the medical title. It was a surgical review journal. It almost looked like a prop, in a position facing Haims, rather than dropped by the reader. Everything was neat. In spite of having said Schmidt was in charge, the scene aroused Hank's curiosity.

He put on a pair of plastic gloves. One bullet hole was present in the head at the right temporo-parietal area—the side of the head. Contact wounds over bone were different in that a rim of black powder was not always obvious around the entrance into the skin—it had to be analyzed in the deeper tissue and bone. An exit wound was not obvious but he needed to be more thorough to confirm it.

Sometimes an exit wound was in the neck or upper chest, even though the entrance was in the head. Bullets did strange things when they tumbled around the inside of the skull. Some he had found even in the intestine. An X-ray of the body before commencing the autopsy reduced the time in locating the slug or pieces of the slug.

A gun was in Haims's right hand with the finger on the trigger. Hank gently tried to move the jaw—early rigor mortis changes started here. Rigor was minimal. The arms and legs were still flaccid; the body still warm. Death was very recent.

Something nagged at him—bothered him. He was trained in this. He should know. What was it?

Something important. Something was not right. Or was it simply an emotional response to Haims's death? He viewed the scene as dispassionately as he could. What was the scene telling him?

Start with the wound. Was it a contact wound; near, intermediate, or a distance shot? What were the characteristics of each? Blood was present on the chair and some had oozed out the back of the head and dried.

That was it! The blood-spatter pattern was incorrect. Gently, Hank moved the head and looked at the occiput—the back of the head. It was definitely foul play. Suicide could be ruled out.

Hank stood back and viewed the entire room, obviously Haims's personal study. It was nicely furnished in the taste of the local interior decorator whose ambiance didn't vary much.

On the floor, a machine copy of an oriental rug was present. A passable copy. A telephone was on a pad which was molded into the library wall. Three walls were covered with books behind glassed doors. Haims disproved of fiction in general. A surgeon's medical practice, he believed, did not allow time for *literary escapism*, as he termed it. The medical books showed signs of honest use. The fourth wall of the room consisted predominately of French doors which opened out into the garden and street.

Hank turned his attention to Mrs. Haims. She was quietly talking to the police officers.

What did he know about her? In the medical community, the wives thought of Mrs. John Haims as a partial recluse. She was not too well-known and often not recognized in town. It was rumored that she devoted herself to the church and to her family, but no one saw her at any of the usual activities.

Hank observed her, trying to do so unobtrusively. She was a fairly pretty woman, small featured, and he judged her to be in her early fifties, although the excessive strain lines on her face made her look much older. A blue robe covered her nightgown. She was dry-eyed, made small body movements, and her voice barely shook with emotion as she answered the detective's questions.

Although her voice and face were quiet, her hands kept wringing small circles around a tightly held handkerchief when she wasn't placing it in the pocket of the blue robe and just as quickly retrieving it.

Monty Catori, the head detective, was interviewing her.

"I don't know what made me look in on the doctor," she said. "He usually comes to bed early because of his surgery schedule. But tonight I fell asleep after reading and woke up and found him."

"How soon did you call us after finding him, ma'am?"

"Right away. Well, actually, I called the ambulance first."

"Yes, ma'am. Anyone else live here with you?"

"My son and daughter. But they're both away at school right now. My other son Jonathan is in California."

"Is that the doctor's gun?"

"I don't know. He has a gun collection but I wouldn't know one from the other. I was always afraid of them—he insisted on keeping them loaded, you know."

"Yes, ma'am. Were there any visitors or anyone expected for an appointment that you know of?"

"No. The doctor usually kept his business meetings at the office or hospital. Anything we did here was entertainment... but not recently."

Her constant referral to Haims as *the doctor* was jarring

to Hank because it was delivered with the same tone one used in referring to the Almighty.

He hadn't heard about entertainment by the Haimses at their home. Could it be some other social group? Haims worked with his referral doctors and friends by reserving space at the local restaurants fairly often, but rarely with his wife present. Haims had invited Corky and himself several times, but Haims's wife had been absent and they were told that she never came.

Monty was a clever detective. Hank had observed his methods before and admired the quiet probing about depression, business debts, enemies, problems with their children or marriage—gently but thoroughly. All the answers to his questions would be carefully written down and within the next few hours, they would be all typed up and ready for signing. The witnesses' signatures were down before they had time to think and rearrange events in their minds.

Almost casually, Monty had her hands checked out for gun powder residue. The chief was still there, quiet, unobtrusive, listening and watching everyone.

"When did Dr. Schmidt say he was going to do the post-mortem, Chief?" Hank asked.

"Said about nine o'clock. That's about four hours from now. You going to be there?" Hank nodded. "See you then." The chief pulled down his cap and left.

When he returned home, it was 5:30 A.M. He stayed downstairs and read a journal until Corky woke up an hour later.

"How did it go?" She was asking the cause of death as she made the coffee.

"Slug went into the right side of his head."

"How horrible."

"Yes." It was—horrible. Just as she said. Yet he felt little emotion.

Pathologists trained themselves not to be bothered about the horrible part of human conditions—blood, vomit, infectious fluids. They had to think and keep thinking when everyone was upset—quietly doing what had to be done, quickly, without emotion. The end result was that they were thought of as cold, forbidding doctors. Devoid of normal emotions. Impervious. Different. Odd. Scary even.

With Haims dead, his problems were over. Span had no reason to continue the attack. Or did he?

Seven

Hank arrived bleary-eyed at the lab in the morning and saw the red light above the door of the morgue was lit, signaling that an autopsy was in progress.

He walked in and saw Schmidt at the sink, washing the instruments and putting them in the stainless steel container for autoclaving.

"Finished?" he said. "A bit early?"

"Yes," said Schmidt. "I've got other work to do."

"What'd you find on Haims?"

"The expected."

"Nothing else?"

"No."

Schmidt looked at Hank antagonistically.

"You had X-rays taken of the head and chest, determined the angle of the handgun, recovered and handled the slug so the markings weren't disturbed and took vitreous fluid from the eyes, hours apart, for estimating the time of death—all this?" Hank knew Schmidt only used internal core temperature and rigor mortis to establish the time of death.

Schmidt hesitated as his eyes flickered back to the body. He didn't reply and turned away. Never mind, Hank thought. You just told me you left out something.

Out loud Hank said, "Better to do it. These things can be come back to haunt you." Schmidt looked away. "Only one slug?"

"Yes."

Hank glanced at the lines of fracture on the occiput, the back of the empty skull plate and at the brain sitting in formalin nestled in a wide-mouthed plastic bucket. Clearly, the slug had tumbled through the brain, leaving a lacerated track much like perforations in vanilla Jell-O. One slug could make a mush of the brain.

"Where was the slug?" asked Hank persistently.

"Brain."

The brain had been removed, leaving a gaping empty hollow in the head. The skin flaps of the scalp draped down from the skull and the dura mater; the thick membrane lining covering the brain surface was loosely hanging on the inside. The lines of fracture on the back and sides of the empty skull plate looked like cracks in an eggshell dropped too many times.

Hank couldn't resist admonishing Schmidt: "Hope you took a lot of pictures and are prepared to explain which event came first: the blow, the gunshot wound, or the poisoning." He had already seen enough to confirm two of those diagnoses. The third, the poison bit, he threw out to Schmidt without evidence.

Schmidt flung the cutting tools into a container. The noise reverberated in the small, cheerless room.

When Hank went back into the laboratory, he was greeted normally. The laboratorians had adjusted. The greetings this time were without hesitation. Yesterday's problems were yesterday's. Today presented a new set of difficulties. Life went on.

Hank began the day's work of bone marrow biopsies, proceeded with the problem blood smears that the techs had placed on his desk, and then finished with the interpretations of the cardiac enzymes and serum electrophoreses—these latter tests were the first to change when a patient was having a heart attack. Two patients he diagnosed as having such attacks: an acute coronary thrombosis or a myocardial infarct.

Time for the coffee break. Hank took his diagnoses and gave them to Ed to review. Ed looked at the papers wordlessly. Better bring it out into the open, Hank thought. "A bit of work for you to look over and initial. Committee's orders."

"Oh. Yes," he replied. "So I've heard." He said nothing more.

Hank looked at Ed expectantly but Ed was not going to say anything else. No sympathy. No embarrassment. Just bald acceptance that Hank's work was to be reviewed. His action spoke volumes. Was he one of the pathologists who felt Hank's diagnoses were criminal?

Hank strolled out to the lab entrance and relaxed by viewing the soft lights, carpeting and greenery in their lobby. The walls were hung with prints from the Metropolitan Museum of Art—mostly Impressionists, American and European. Hank had brightened up the lab waiting room in an attempt to relieve the sterile atmosphere, at least in this corner of the hospital. It pleased him to view his own oasis like a contented beast, even for a few minutes.

Bill Enzer walked in.

"When's the post?" he asked Hank.

"Dr. Schmidt's case. Already done," Hank replied.

Enzer's eyes registered surprise, then a little anger. He liked to be present at autopsies on any problem cases involving well-known individuals to make sure nothing was overlooked. This was always assumed as the chief's ongoing request and Hank always waited for him until he could be present.

"You'll have to check with Dr. Schmidt," Hank said. "The organs were all out of the body and in the bucket when I arrived about seven this morning."

The chief frowned, then spun around and headed for Dr. Schmidt's office.

"Hold it," said Hank. "He's now in my office."

Chief only nodded and turned in the right direction.

He was back almost immediately. His face was red and frown lines were obvious. Whatever the discussion was with Schmidt, it made the chief most unhappy.

Eight

Every morning, Hank made a point to visit a room off surgery where the physicians gathered before the day's work. The room was furnished with coffee, juice and pastries. Pop-corn was a recent obsession and the smell pervaded the rooms. It was here that complaints about the lab were often aired and easily resolved before they became problems. Most were justified in the minds of the attendings, but almost always the lab was blamed needlessly.

Today was Monday and no different. Hank was nailed immediately about a report that had been delayed. A quick phone call settled the difficulty. The specimen had arrived Friday evening, and because the analysis could only be made on a specimen kept in a frozen state, it had been held in their freezer until Monday morning. Physicians wanted instant results on everything—a normal reaction.

No one mentioned Hank's reduced status and Hank didn't expect them to do so. Each physician had enough problems to handle all day. The hierarchy in the laboratory did not concern them in the least, only that accurate work was performed. Steve Short, the urologist who had been at the ad hoc meeting, looked startled when he saw Hank and he got up to pour himself a cup of coffee in the corner.

Quietly bantering, not missing anything, was Tim Hawkes, in his usual spot. He, too, kept in contact with the staff by making the off-surgery room a place for a routine daily visit.

Satisfied that the situation was normal, Hank left the hospital for the Bolli, located in downtown Red Wolf.

At the Bolli, he was a member of a coffee group that had an uncanny sense of knowing what was going on in the city. Over and over, he had acquired information, all under the category of gossip, certainly, that was almost always correct and useful.

The group seemed to know who was getting fired, promoted, or allowed to resign; where the new streets were to be built or roads resurfaced; and the more amusing details of domestic difficulties. Even the latter was of interest and filed away so that no one would make a stupid error of inquiring about the health of someone's wife when they had been divorced for months.

The discussions were freewheeling and more on the level of a fraternity. Practical jokes were the norm. Any show of embarrassment caused the others to roar with laughter and the storyteller was applauded.

The actual truth was unimportant and if the victim tried to protest his innocence, all the better.

The day before had been a birthday party for Riggers, the car dealer. Two flat, rounded pieces of sponge had been covered with chocolate and several candles placed on the "cake." Riggers had been almost teary-eyed at the sentiment until he tried to cut it. He began to complain about the blunt knife and was immediately handed another with apologies. When the second knife wouldn't cut either, he realized something was wrong. Then he threw down the knife and swore. Naturally, "chocolate cake" would be a special item of discussion for the week.

Dr. Haims's death was being discussed when Hank entered and poured himself a cup of coffee.

Tom Pinch turned his coffee cup around and said, "A lot of folks often speculated why he wasn't done away with years ago..." He looked up just then, saw Hank and stopped.

"Sorry, Doc." he said. "You know how we like to run on about doctors and lawyers—always open season on them, you know."

Hank shrugged, smiled and nodded. He wanted to talk to Riggers, the local Pontiac dealer who had been having some chest pain and blackouts, and try to convince him to have a checkup. His symptoms were clearly those of high blood pressure.

Hank sat next to Riggers in the booth and began easily enough. Then he began to cajole and then humorously threaten by citing the consequences. It was no use.

"Humor me, Riggers, and repeat back what I just said," asked Hank.

"...That the pushy way I work, my blood pressure is going to keep going up and down, up and down, until finally it's going to stay up. Then I'm going to either clot up a blood vessel or blow it out in the brain and cause a stroke. Also that I'm going to have heart and kidney problems."

"Good. You *were* listening."

"I understand what you said." Riggers's face was earnest as he explained. "But I want to live the way I'm living—all stops out—and if something happens, then it happens!"

Hank shrugged and shook his head. "Well, you're an intelligent person and if that's what you want, then that's what you want."

Twenty minutes had gone by and Hank was heading out the door when the police chief, oddly restrained in his greeting, walked in.

It had been four days since the autopsy on Dr. Haims. The newspapers had reported it as "under investigation" and were inquiring, suspicious that they weren't being completely informed.

"Need to talk to you about some personal things regarding Dr. Haims. Drop down this afternoon at the station, will you?" The chief seemed to grunt the invitation.

"Sure. Two-thirty all right?"

"Fine."

This was a switch. The chief always came to the hospital for information. Never the other way around. Something else was brewing.

• • •

Two-thirty came quickly.

The police aide who had been there for ages recognized him and said, "They're waiting for you in the back."

Chief Enzer, Monty and a stenographer were in the room. An interrogation—not an informal meeting.

"Doc," said the chief laconically, "you have anything against our asking you some questions?"

Hank nodded acceptance.

"Your name, occupation and city of residence?"

"Hank Whipple. Pathologist. Red Wolf."

"Name of hospital you practice in? How long?

"St. Mary's. About ten years."

"Any problems with other physicians?"

"The usual, almost always resolved." Hank began to suspect where the questions were leading.

"Tell us about your relationship with Dr. Haims—did you like him?"

"He's on the staff at St. Mary's. Performs most of the general surgery."

"You haven't told us whether you liked or disliked him."

"Obviously, I have...had to get along with him. He performed the most surgery and therefore sent us the most surgical specimens. He wasn't easy to chat with," said Hank.

Monty smiled. "Can we take that to mean...if you had your druthers, you wouldn't?"

"That's right."

"How did you lose your job as director? Who promotes and who fires?" They had been talking to someone. Hopefully someone without a jaundiced eye.

"In some hospitals, often no one wants the job because of the added responsibility. In this hospital, it's a desirable job with increased pay—a salaried job. The administrator scales the position."

"Does he first get the opinions of the other doctors in the hospital?"

"If he's wise, he does. This administrator is wise," replied Hank.

"How about demotions? Same thing?"

"No...not really."

The chief broke in, "You hesitated. Does that mean the administrator didn't consult the other doctors before demoting you?"

"That's right."

"Did you ask to be demoted or was it done for a reason?"

There it was. How was he going to explain it without appearing paranoid or self-serving? He said, "Dr. Haims was able to use his influence and cause the demotion."

"Did this have anything to do with your being up for problems with your diagnoses?"

"No. This was before the ad hoc committee met." Hank could feel himself beginning to burn. Someone had leaked all the confidential details. It was a jaundiced eye, after all.

"Tell us about how these committees work. Exactly what did they complain about?"

Hank described the various committees in the hospital. They looked bored as he talked—they were waiting for something else.

Finishing with hospital policies, the questions concerned the various character traits of the physicians. Psychopaths? How would Hank know? Were they checking him for paranoid thoughts?

Hank asked permission to use their phone and explain his prolonged absence to the laboratory. He returned to the chair.

"Then we take it that you disliked Dr. Haims—even hated him for causing you to lose your job."

"'Dislike' would be a fair word," said Hank.

"Enough dislike...hate...to kill him?"

Hank grimaced. "No!...so that's where you're leading!"

Chief Enzer's face had retreated behind an official mask. The policeman he had known for years was performing his duty. Hank reeled at the thought. He was a suspect in Haims's murder!

The questions continued and now revolved around when Hank saw the deceased John Haims last. With each answer, their faces retreated behind official masks. He told himself it was their job not to believe anyone, but it didn't soften the anxiety.

The stenographer held up her hand to stop the questioning until she had changed the recording tape.

"Where did you say you went the late night or early morning when Haims died?" Monty asked.

Hank explained how he had taken a long walk alone. Not a usual thing. No. His wife vouch for him? No, she was asleep. Did he see anyone who could confirm his whereabouts? No. Monty and the chief just looked at him. Expressionless.

Hank told himself that it was not a personal insult. Even clergymen of advanced years were not exempt from a police officer's cynicism. It came with the territory, just like his own territory. Just because Hank had worked with the police for years did not exempt him from suspicion. Just the same, it still hurt to be considered a possible murder suspect. The silence continued.

Finally, Monty said, "Is there anything you left out that you would like to tell us?"

A fishing question. What could he say? Hank shook his head.

"That's it then for the time being," said the chief. "We'll be in touch, as the saying goes."

Hank got up and left. The room spun slightly as he walked into the street. He was a suspect in the murder of Dr. Haims!

Why? Haims must have told a number of people about their confrontation—twisting the details and conversation to his advantage. What had Hank said that could be construed as a death threat?

It was true that he *had* threatened Haims—an indirect threat involving a loss of status and livelihood. But the Haimses of the world were able to bounce back and always surface elsewhere with a slightly different twist to their scams.

Hank went back to the lab for any messages.

The new secretary was flustered and apologetic. She had signed for a registered letter addressed to Hank. Was that all right? She looked at Hank anxiously. Of course.

The registered letter was from the ad hoc tissue surgery committee. Span said it was mailed Wednesday. Today was Monday.

It contained a laundry list of anatomical diagnoses Hank had made, together with copies of the reports. Hank expected more than the dozen disputed. They were varied cases: Pap smears, breast carcinomas, malignant lymphomas, metastatic tumors, and the like. There was no review of his diagnoses by any other pathologists enclosed. Hank checked the envelope again.

Nothing. Since the cases could not be judged by any physician other than a pathologist, Hank wondered who or whom the committee found to review the diagnoses. In any case, now he had what he needed to prepare his own defense.

Hank tried to remember what Fuller Span had said about the review of his work. He had assumed the consultant pathologist's comments would be included with the reports. What was it that Span said? Hank asked himself. Did he say it would be included?

Dr. Span's number was busy. When Hank did reach the office, Dr. Span was reportedly gone. Hank left a message.

He made excuses to Corky and remained at the lab. He looked up the records on the reports he had received in the mail. There was no fiddling with the words. Those were his exact diagnoses. He pulled the glass slides containing slices of surgical tissue.

An hour later, he had finished his review. Hank felt much better. Only three were in gray areas of interpretation. Two other diagnoses were made without being made aware of the clinical findings. Inflammatory dermatoses of the skin were always difficult without any background information. To the clinician who had the patient's history, the diagnosis was reduced to a few possibilities. Insufficient information was a fact of their practice—as it was for the radiologist. It was often impossible to reach the clinician for more information, so a number of probable diagnoses were offered. These were termed "differential diagnoses."

The Pap smears were correctly diagnosed. He felt secure in those since he had kept up on the latest cytology seminars and had completed the last workshop only a few months ago.

Hank went home satisfied that he could defend himself. In the morning, he would ship the slides and reports to Seattle and have two consultant pathologists evaluate them.

An hour late for dinner, Corky hurriedly said, "Tell the children you're home."

She seemed so relaxed and happy that he decided not to mention anything about the letter from the quality assurance committee or the interrogation at the police station. Instead, for the first time in weeks, he was able to push his problems aside and relax for the evening.

But in spite of the rekindling of confidence in himself, Hank slept poorly. He found himself going over and over each report. When he stopped thinking about the reports, he began reviewing the interrogation in the police station. He was a murder suspect.

This type of thing he couldn't discuss with Corky. She'd only get worried and there was little she could do anyway. This was his bailiwick.

Nine

The next morning he was again in the surgical lounge. It was filled with doctors and camaraderie.

"Are you coming to Keith's party?" The questioner was Billups, an anesthesiologist.

"What party?" asked Hank, startled.

"I'm sure you're invited—everyone usually is—even pathologists."

"Might. When is it?"

"Oh, it's posted around here somewhere. Take a look." With that, Billups disappeared out the hall into an operating room.

How unusual that life went on in spite of a surgeon's

death, thought Hank. Before he had time to muse over this, Keith Gray came in.

"Party?" Hank asked.

"Oh...yes," he replied. "Darlene and I had it planned for several weeks. Hope you can come. Bring Corky." He paused for an afterthought. "Poor timing on our part with Haims's death and we hope no one takes it wrong, but the food will spoil if we keep it any longer and we have no place to put it."

Hank shrugged and made a noncommittal remark. The room was now filled with physicians. Many of them did not perform surgery or even assist but needed the stimulation of contact and discussion of patients and their problems. Interspersed between talk of sports, cars and medical practice problems, came the solving of medical problems and offhand "curbstone" consultations.

Tim nodded at Hank when their eyes met as though nothing had happened. Tim began talking sports and offering bets but no one would acknowledge his offers because of the complicated method that he used—two or three teams together in one bet. He almost always won.

Sam Sager had a one-liner joke: "The difference between a sperm and a lawyer—the sperm has a chance at being a human being." Sam was warm to everyone regardless. His hands were huge and he referred to them as "Sam's hams"—displaying them proudly, whenever anyone took notice, explaining they were the result of years of working on construction to get through school.

Sam had gone through the same school as John Haims— they were of the same religion as well—but the similarities in personality and style stopped there. No one excluded Hank in any conversation but no one included him, either. He had become a questionable entity even after ten years of practice there. A slow build-up of reputation and an immediate shunning if any question of ability or impropriety occurred. Well, it would build back up quickly enough.

Back at the lab, Hank reflected that, except for the members of the ad hoc committee, the other doctors reacted with normally.

He stopped in front of his former office. Schmidt's autopsy dictation on Dr. Haims should be out and rough-typed.

Sure enough. The draft was on the desk. Since they all routinely read each other's work, Hank paused and picked up the material.

An autopsy begins at the scene of the crime—not at the autopsy table. Every bit of information mattered—small things: observations by mailmen, delivery men and neighbors; even conversations between on-scene investigators might bring out factors which changed the entire thrust of the autopsy procedure and subsequent diagnoses.

Scanning the double-spaced page, it was a surprise to read Schmidt's summary. Much had been left out in the description including blood spatter, angle of the trajectory, skull fracture lines and removal of pieces of tissue from around the entrance wound. Schmidt, although untrained in forensic work, nevertheless prided himself on describing important details. How could he have left out descriptions of several organs?

"Meet with your approval?" The voice behind was Schmidt's.

"No."

"But then, nothing ever does, does it?"

There was no use replying.

"Will someone explain this to me?"

The voice came from Steve French, an astute doctor in family practice.

"Yes," they both replied simultaneously. Schmidt swiftly

moved and cut Hank off by blocking the doorway with his back.

Hank turned and picked up the autopsy protocol again. Some gall bladder calculi. Congestion of organs. Rare plaques of arteriosclerosis in the larger blood vessels. Dr. Haims was fastidious about his diet and it showed. Stomach contents. Nothing dictated. The internal temperature of the body was taken. Early rigor mortis had been noted in the jaw at the scene and the increase at the autopsy table. Seemingly complete, to the practiced eye, it was surprisingly sketchy. Verbose, with large amounts of verbiage, but in terms of real useful content for forensics, it was a dud.

"Thank you. See you two around!" called Steve French over Schmidt's shoulder to Hank. Steve, a sensitive doctor, noted the body block and was going out of his way to acknowledge his friendliness to Hank. One person like that made up for a lot of callous people.

Hank continued to look at the completed reports on the autopsy. It was mandatory to run barbiturate, cocaine, opium, benzdiazepine, cannabis and other tests on the urine in all forensic cases. There was no report. An estimated time of death was not present.

"Schmidt," Hank said, "this is not a forensic autopsy. You've done a hospital-death type of evaluation. This can't be turned out without the routines of probable time of death, complete organ descriptions and picture explanation of the external wound entrance and the micros in that area."

"Keep out of this!" Schmidt exclaimed, grabbing the draft sheets. "This is *my* report. You're not the only one who thinks he can do forensic work!"

His face became even more furious. "Besides, you're the one under investigation for incompetence. Not me!"

Hank was caught by surprise at the loud outburst. It was

unusual for Schmidt to allow his temper to explode in the lab. Naturally, everyone could hear him.

As an assistant pathologist, Schmidt had been a model of politeness. Not once could Hank remember Schmidt raising his voice during that time.

Hank went back to his desk. If Schmidt didn't want criticism of the autopsy, so be it.

He had hardly sat down when the oncologists came in to review their bone marrows and chemical reports.

Oncologists dealt daily with the worst in life—cancer. They worked in a world of deep anguish and continuous pain, and became expert at relieving pain from various origins by trying to reduce the progression of the malignant tumor. Today they were looking any ray of hope—any improvement in the chemical reports or biopsies for their patients.

"Another myeloma," grimaced the oncologist. He had just finished his training and was still emotionally vulnerable. "I suspected it."

"Yes," replied Hank evenly.

The electrophoretic pattern had shown a monoclonal spike in the gamma fraction. This was a test in which a drop of serum was placed in an electric field, causing the serum proteins of spread out. Staining the material and placing it in an analyzer instrument ordinarily produced curves, but instead of curves, this time one revealed a "monoclonal spike," which usually meant multiple myeloma—a bone marrow cancer. A bone marrow aspiration and biopsy confirmed the diagnosis.

"Third this month," he said to Hank.

"Fourth, actually," Hank replied.

"Whose case?" The oncologist was curious.

"Out of town."

In one way, Hank realized he had the easy part—the

diagnosis. The hard part was telling the patient, or deciding against that, telling the spouse or relatives. This disease was one of the many afflictions of middle and old age when the immune system began to deteriorate.

The last marrow smears and biopsies were still next to the microscope. "A forty-five-year-old male. Anemia. Malaise. Night sweats. Marked loss of weight unrelated to food intake." All this was typical of any cancer. The triad of anemia, low platelets and excessively high white blood count meant leukemia.

Acute leukemia could now be helped. The cell chromosomes were analyzed and the exact area of chromosomal translocation, duplication, addition or simple deletion, would be reported. From these facts, the progress of the leukemia could be ascertained.

Hank looked at the person's name. It was a small town so Hank knew him. He would soon see more of him as time went on as he came into the laboratory more and more often. Hopefully, his chromosomes were such that the prognosis would be favorable with chemotherapy or, failing that, a bone marrow transplant would be palliative or perhaps curative.

Hank looked at the bare wall and sighed. How small his problems were compared to what others had—even as a murder suspect. Surely the police weren't serious about that. Wasn't his main thrust to keep his job? His wife Corky would back him.

Still, his problems were nothing compared to an outlook of living with a cancer that slowly and painfully sucked out the marrow of existence.

Ten

"Dr. Whipple, can I see you for a moment?" The almost unobtrusive voice of Darrel Sims, chemistry supervisor. "Well, I might as well tell you of a problem," Darrel said. "We're not supposed to give out the test results to the patients. There's one patient who demands to know his testosterone test numbers."

"You mean Cliff Evers?" Hank saw him waiting in the lobby.

Cliff broke horses for a living but was available for other work at the Roundup Grounds. Wrangling thousand-pound animals was tough physical labor. Perhaps that was why he had undergone a double hernia repair and hydrocele repairs on both sides, unfortunately ending up with the abscesses of both testicles.

At the Roundup Grounds, Hank decided to talk to Cliff about it in the hospital setting.

"Yes. He's panicked with the low results."

"Apparently he's been getting the results before. Why do you consider it a problem now?" asked Hank.

"As usual, Dr. Haims does not want patients to receive results, but Cliff is related to a tech on the night shift who was sympathetic enough to slip him the results." Darrel half-expected a reprimand but knew better.

Hank sat back in his chair. "Well…you know how I feel about test results. A patient who pays for them should have the right to receive them. It's the attending physician's lookout to interpret them or have the pathologist do it."

Darrel looked embarrassed. "It gets worse. Dr. Haims lied to him. I guess I can say that now that he's dead. He told Cliff there was nothing to worry about and that everything would be all right."

"And gave him the usual 'I'm busy' brushoff," mused Hank. "But Cliff knew different—how long since his surgery?"

"About six or eight months."

"And now he is having all kinds of changes, including mental ones. I suppose he turned him over to Dr. Span, who is playing with low-impact antibiotics." Hank sighed. Cliff's atrophied testicles were producing minimal male hormone and his sex drive was markedly diminished or gone. He had to be frightened. And angry.

All body hormones have a definite mental influence whenever there was a lack or overabundance. Agitated depression was too commonly overlooked and the patient was labeled as neurotic. Surgeons were the worst offenders in follow-ups on patients—they were trained to cut and felt their jobs were done when the wound healed.

Darrel interrupted his thoughts. "His wife has left him."

"She married a macho cowboy and now... He's about twenty-six years old. Right?"

Darrel nodded. "And no children. I can see where he'd be real upset."

The circulation had stopped in his feet so Hank got up, shifted his weight and went outside to the corridor. Cliff Evers was looking at the wall in the lobby. Hank resolved to stop equivocating and help this cowboy.

The unwritten rule said one doctor never interfered with another's patient unless requested to do so by the patient. Well, that unwritten rule would have to go in this case. Cliff needed guidance and he couldn't keep on watching him endure and endure and wait for someone like Span to finally give up and send him in the right direction.

Cliff Evers was sitting, staring straight ahead—a contrast to the other patients who were reading or herding their children about the lobby. His ever-present cowboy hat was rarely removed.

"Cliff. Let's talk." Hank motioned with his head toward his private office. This time he wouldn't give up easily. Too much depended upon it. Reluctantly Cliff got up and followed Hank into his office.

Hospitals intimidated everybody. The walls, the floors, the important bustling of hospital employees, the abrupt and persistent voices paging faceless names over the loudspeaker—all contributing to the impersonal. Cliff looked at him warily.

"You already know about your lab results. Your hormone level is down. You need a doctor who works with people in your condition."

Cliff stared and partly glared at him without speaking.

Hank persisted. "Would you let me call someone who can help you?"

Cliff nodded. Good! At least there was an admission of the problem.

"I'm calling a doctor, a woman doctor, so don't get upset and turn macho. She's a specialist in something called endocrinology—which is a fancy term for someone who checks out how the different hormones are working in a person. Too much can harm. Too little can harm. She will analyze, pinpoint the problem and balance everything out."

"You want me to go see this woman doctor?"

"Yes."

"I've never been to a woman doctor. Will she want to check me all over?"

"All over."

"Everything?"

"Yes. Everything!" Hank grinned in spite of himself.

Cliff thought a moment, looked up and caught the grin.

"Better get used to it, Cliff. Half of the doctors now graduating are women. Sooner or later, you're going to need one."

Cliff nodded hesitantly. "Yeah. I guess."

Hank reached back to the desk, flipped through the roto-file and dialed a number. Ordinarily, he would have asked a secretary to call, but with Cliff, it was best to maintain the personal and keep things confidential.

"Jane? Hank here. Would you work a patient into your schedule as soon as possible? Personal favor. Thanks."

Hank turned to Cliff. "This Wednesday. Eleven A.M. Can you make it?" Cliff nodded. Hank confirmed the appointment.

"You guarantee she'll help me?"

"Yes."

Cliff stared at Hank. "Why didn't that other cutting doctor or his pal do what you just did?"

"I don't know. It doesn't matter. What matters is for you to get back on a normal keel."

Cliff shifted uneasily in his chair and pulled down his hat. "Why can't you do what she's going to do? You're a doctor."

"I could, but I'd have to see you over and over and keep on top of your problem. A culture is necessary to make sure what antibiotic will kill the infection. It's not a one-shot deal like giving you some penicillin. Then, the hormone takes balancing and balancing takes time. Besides, I don't like you that much and seeing you too often would make me puke!"

Cliff got up. A grin on the usually impassive face. "I won't forget this, you know."

"All I did was make a phone call. You owe me nothing."

"Yeah. Right. One phone call. I know what you just did."

Hermy, the immunochemistry supervisor, was waiting outside Hank's door. It had to be a pressing problem, otherwise, she would have gone away and returned later.

Cliff got up and gratefully stuck out his hand.

Hermy shouldered her way in as Cliff left and presented several test results which were skewed. Computers analyzed blood accurately but now and then there was a glitch. Their in-house quality control had caught the glitch. It would take work to straighten out the problem and until then, no testing would be performed on that instrument. That was part of his job.

They discussed the problem and decided it had to be the hardware. A call to the instrument manufacturer sufficed. A new hardware board was being Fed-Expressed that morning. Finished, Hank walked outside and drove to the

Roundup Grounds.

He hated the idea of leaving Red Wolf. Hank had been a Rodeo director now for five years—the offer of membership was also a vote that he had been accepted by this small community. It felt good to smell the horses and barns. The earthy conversation of the ranchers, cowboys and farmers was a welcome relief.

Next to the breaking corral, Lou Gavins, the groundskeeper, was showing off his race horse Lucky. Lou liked the word "Lucky" and would use any product using that word. Lucky beer, Lucky aftershave, Lucky cigarettes, Lucky anything—Lou would buy.

"Are you still trying to sell that bag of bones, Lou? He won't bring five cents a pound at the cannery!"

Someone else joined in. "Naw! He's going to put him in the one hundred dollar claiming race and stick somebody with him."

Lou always thought slowly. The idea of selling his horse for dog food unsettled him and he shook his head. His over-large straw hat bounced in the wind. He decided to ignore both jibes.

"Going to win big in Spokane next week—he's looking great!" Lou smiled proudly at the horse who was standing quietly.

"How about Miss Mustard?" asked Cliff Evers.

Lou's smile broadened. "She always wins. You know that!"

"Claiming race?"

"Claiming race? No!" Lou looked shocked at the cowboy. "Hell no! I wouldn't enter her in a claiming race! Ain't enough money in the world to make me give her up!" Pride at the thought of his favorite horse caused him to straighten up his spine and stand tall. He tilted his head back so that his eyes slanted downward beneath his large straw hat.

The group had found Lou's vulnerable spot again. "Seems to me you have a little trouble cornering the truth," began one of the men leaning on the fence.

"Why?" Lou sputtered. "It's the God's truth..."

Hank walked away. That conversation was good for at least fifteen minutes. He'd heard the same bait snapped up by Lou over and over. But in the end, someone would purchase a percentage of Lou's racehorse just to share in Lou's excitement about racing.

Cliff Evers was taking part so at least temporarily he was out of his depression.

Hank looked down the barn area. There they were as usual. His three children were sitting on the fence, talking while their mother was brushing the horse.

"Why is it all mothers think they have to do the grooming?" he asked Corky.

He found a brush and began helping. After fourteen years of marriage, she still looked as young and pretty as ever. The hair on her head was wet and the freckles stood out on her face which was flushed from the exertion. Her once white tennis shoes were muddied. He was a lucky man.

She looked up, smiled and started to speak. Hank stopped her. "I know. I know. The children don't do a good enough job." She continued to smile. They had gone through this enough times.

She was brushing the second horse that they had ever owned. Old Doc was a gelding of indeterminate age. After he had been acquired, they found he had a fungus infection of the skin. Being new to the horse world, the Whipples bought some medication from the vet and applied it all over his body.

The next day, Old Doc wouldn't come out of his stall and when he was finally caught, haltered and led out, he pulled away suddenly and ran from them. He had taken one look at the bottle of medicine in their hand and bolted. For the first time they read the instructions: "Dilute one ounce in a gallon of water." They had applied the concentrated solution and, in their innocence, had tortured his entire body. No wonder he fled!

Hank watched her continue to brush Old Doc, then coaxed the children to bridle and saddle their mother's horse. Hank went and got his own.

Corky had purchased their first horse for Hank. It was a gentle ranch horse that would not win any halter show prizes. She named him, aptly, Crummy, but he needed very little guidance and was such a willing animal in spite of being old, that Hank found it important to spare him.

Crum was loose with the other horses but came in on call. His greeting was always the same—placing the front of his head on Hank's chest and shoving gently. Their game.

Once in a while, Crum would simply place his head on Hank's chest and leave it there. Hank learned to interpret this as meaning he was not feeling good. Old age did that to you. He wished he knew how old Crum was. No horse-trader told the truth. On those off days, Hank brushed him down gently, taking lots of time, and fed him an extra amount of grain and vitamins. If he had been kept in a stall that day, they did a slow walk and a light trot up and down the grounds only. The mild exercise seemed to revive Crum because often the next time, Crum usually felt full of energy and they rode for hours.

They had a satisfying relationship. Horse and man. Each enjoying and protecting the other. It was such a relief not to have a horse that ran for the barn as soon as it could. Barn-sour animals were a misery—as were horses that bit, kicked or tried to run away with you.

Crum preferred the hackmore instead of the bridle and bit. The hackamore looked deceptively simple but wasn't because a pull on the reins compressed the horse's nose. In the wrong hands, it could be more painful than a bit in the mouth.

Hank's saddle was purchased at a bargain from Dr. Haims. Those were fun days when they rode together. Haims was different then. Or acted differently, anyway. Haims's children became teenagers with teenagers' problems, and although he continued to have the desire, Haims never had the time for riding. After that, he explained it as "family trouble." It was never referred to again, since Haims sold all his equipment and horses.

Corky saw to it that their family had time together. They tried to keep pretty much on a schedule of Mondays, Wednesdays, Fridays for riding and Tuesdays, Thursdays and Saturdays for his athletic club activities. An hour a day for physical work. It swept the mind of cobwebs. Simple, but it seemed to work.

The children decided to stay at the grounds and play. Hank and Corky climbed the hill behind the grounds on their horses and looked down at the Snake and Clearwater Rivers. Corky's cheeks bloomed on every ride—it was one of his pleasures to note her physical response to her favorite activity.

When they returned to the Roundup Grounds, one of the Rodeo directors, Riggers, the Pontiac dealer, was there and, while putting Crum away, they discussed the board meeting at the local hotel. The Rodeo parade needed to be worked on, for one thing. A decision of who would go to Denver and sign up the clowns and acts was another.

With schoolboy logic, he found he was delaying his return to the hospital. Had he known what was yet to come, he would have been even more averse.

Eleven

When he arrived at the hospital he found the dictated reports typed and ready for signing. His timing was good. While initialing the reports, he found someone looking over his shoulder.

It was Dr. Span. "Where's Dr. Schmidt?" he snapped. "Did he check the work you're doing?"

Hank felt the hot blood rushing to his face. About to reply, he cautioned himself to relax. "Who were the pathologists who labeled my work 'criminal'?" he asked. A question for a question. Even as he asked, he knew Span would not reply.

Span exhaled, mumbled something under his breath

about seeing Schmidt, turned and went down the hall. Hank finished signing the reports. It was now late afternoon.

Early-morning surgery required Hank's presence—not the late afternoon when Ed took over and things simmered down. The lobby area was filling and emptying with patients who were to have surgery tomorrow and needed a blood work-up.

Schmidt's form blocked the doorway. "I've noticed that you're absent a lot during the afternoon."

"Hour and a half every day."

"Suppose someone needed you right then? Since I'm responsible for the lab, I've got to be fair to all."

"I'm on the beeper and there are three other pathologists available."

"Just the same, I've decided that all of us should punch in and punch out—just as the lab techs do."

"Go ahead. Just remember, I come in a half-hour early and take no lunch hour. That makes up for the time away."

"It doesn't look good for you to be seen at the Rodeo Grounds and at the local gym in the middle of the work day."

"Well, Schmidt, I've been doing this for years and will continue. Get lost!"

"Am I to understand you refuse to use a time card?"

"Absolutely."

Schmidt spun around and left.

The day's work over, Hank almost collided at the exit with the administrator. They nodded to each other amiably, but somewhat coolly. Schmidt probably had informed him of his refusal with the time clock. Previously, Tim and he would have chatted about general things, enjoying each other's chatter, but not this time. He watched Tim hurry away and felt the loss.

The next few days passed quickly. He had to try to forget he was under suspicion and keep mentally occupied.

Corky, knowing only the hospital problems, suggested a common-sense approach. "Stay pleasant," she said, "and they'll appreciate you for what you are. And stay on the job. Taking an extended leave—that would be the worst thing you could do."

It was difficult for her role as a spectator, to hear problems and yet not be able to interact within the hospital atmosphere. But her advice, probably naive on the surface, was basically on target. Quitting *would* be the easy way out.

Breakfast time was the hour they talked about their children and the children's problems.

"Amy, your math isn't going well. What's wrong?"

"Nothing. I hate it," she said.

"You know it's important. Can I help?"

"No. I just don't like it."

From her gaze out the window, Hank could see she was going to shut him out. Would she be more receptive at another time?

He looked over at Max, who had just been voted the most popular boy in school.

"Your grades are mediocre overall, Max. Why?"

"All my friends have the same grades, Dad. No one but parents pays attention to grades."

"What help do you need?"

"None. I can do better if I want. We're too busy with sports," Max said.

"Just the same—"

"Leave it, Dad. Don't make me a weirdo. I'm all right. Really." How much should they interfere? Corky shook her head at him silently.

"Marj?"

"Am I next?" grinned Marjorie.

"Yes." Marj was the hardest because she would agree with whatever you said and then do as she pleased. All with a smile.

"Find a new chum since your last friend moved away?"

"No, but I will." She was carefully maintaining a nonchalant air. Marj had Amy and Max, so having a friend was not the most paramount factor in her life. The children left for school.

"Don't forget the party. Tonight," Hank said.

Corky gave him a stricken look. "I don't know if I can go—"

"We must go," he said. "It's one of those necessary events. Especially now."

"But there's so much I have to do here."

"There's never enough time." Hank imitated Corky's voice.

"It's true!"

"I know it's true," said Hank, "but not going would be tantamount to an admission of guilt. I'm quoting from the philosophy of Corky Whipple."

"We'll go," sighed Corky, "but I have a feeling something unpleasant is going to happen."

Twelve

At work, the day went uneventfully. Friday evening arrived and they left for the party.

Keith's home was large, modern, with solid oak timbers in the ceilings and walls and oak flooring throughout, all stained a light color. The windows were leaded and several were of stained glass. A grand piano, matching the oak floors and walls, stood in the middle of the large living room which boasted of a cathedral ceiling.

The party must have begun earlier because it was in full swing when they arrived and the noise was deafening. Many of the guests had imbibed a goodly amount of alcohol.

"Welcome! Pathological ones! Pickle your corpses!" shouted one.

"It's faster if you take out your brain and pickle it first—saves time and wear and tear on the gut!" shouted another.

Hank was cheered at the tone of the raucous greetings. Almost everyone was from St. Mary's or was prominent in town and recognizable. Some spouses weren't there; some he had never met. New doctors seemed to flow into town now, whereas ten years previously, a new doctor was such a rare event that parties were given as a special introduction. Red Wolf was the type of small town they came to now for refuge, hoping to save their offspring from the crime and drug-scene problems of the large cities.

Keith was holding forth about his favorite subject: jogging. He had been in several iron-man type of events and had successfully completed them. The Boston Marathon was the last event in which he had participated—this one would make it the fifth time—and he was discussing the qualifications in order to participate.

"Doctors don't have to undergo the same physical exam that other runners do. They're generally glad to have us sign up, hoping, I suppose, that we'll stop and help someone having trouble and take care of them until the rescue squad comes. They even give physicians special green tags for identification."

Keith continued with a loud, self-deprecating laugh. "The problem is that we're all so competitive in this race, we'll step over a fallen competitor and keep going, glad there's one less guy to beat out."

"And maybe stomp on him on the way?" someone asked, happy to tease Keith.

"If it was shorter to go over him than around, then sure!" exclaimed Keith, twirling his drink and smiling at the thought of shocking his listeners. "Anything to beat your previous time."

Everyone laughed. Someone with a better memory spoke up. "Then how come you stopped to help someone who collapsed? You came in at the end of the race with the stragglers!"

"Well..." Keith looked down at his drink, temporarily at a loss for words. "No one was stopping so I thought I'd have a look."

All of them knew Keith would be most unlikely to leave someone who was sick or in difficulty. Medicine was lucky to have such a kind and considerate person as a member.

The Whipples found themselves with drinks in their hands which tasted good and were well-made. The party was smoothly organized and as a result, the party was going well. Keith's wife, Darlene, was an outgoing reddish-blonde, aware of good clothes and coiffure. She was slim, dressed in a white, gauze affair with a plunging neckline adorned by the ever present gold locket she wore around her neck.

Darlene carried herself with an air of confidence, secure in her secondary role at the party. Keith handled everything at his parties and spared her all the details by having the house professionally cleaned and catered, which was unusual.

In Red Wolf, people usually brought a covered dish to a party—even though everyone could easily afford the food and drinks or catering. This quaint but homey practice would soon go by the wayside as the town's population increased and became citified.

In a town that had so many out of work or in low-paying jobs, it was wise to keep a low profile. The ranchers and cattlemen were never ostentatious. Physicians who spent their money for grown-up toys that were readily visible were frowned upon and lost patients. Keith didn't have to worry about that, since his patients had little choice once they had chosen a surgeon. The anesthesiology group had been organized by Keith and covered both local hospitals and a fifty-mile radius. All surgeons preferred Keith for any difficult case, even though his colleagues were very competent.

Watching, Hank couldn't help feel some professional envy. Keith had charisma. He was sensitive to the needs of others and found the time to be present at weddings and other important events.

The entire surgical nursing crew and surgeons seemed to be there, broken up into groups, laughing and telling stories of their most recent case problems. With the exception of Dr. Haims, of course. No one seemed to mention him. How quickly, even a dominating surgeon, faded from a scene.

"I understand you did the autopsy on Dr. Haims."

Hank turned his gaze from the room to find himself staring into the eyes of Keith's wife, Darlene.

Surprised, he hesitated. "No, I was at the scene. It was performed by Dr. Schmidt."

"Oh," she said. "I overheard your name mentioned in regard to his death and assumed you had performed the post."

"No." He certainly couldn't bring himself to say he was a suspect in the murder. Then for the sake of conversation, he asked, "Did you know him well?"

Surprisingly, she hesitated again and her hand went to the locket around her neck. "No, not really. We never socialized. He never drank or really partied, you know."

Everyone knew Dr. Haims gave only the required gifts and entertainment at the local restaurant as in a business sense, and they were probably accepted in the same sense: a deductible tax expense.

Work schedules had been changed for Haims's benefit,

however. Since his religious beliefs involved no work from sundown Friday until midnight Saturday; Sunday became a regular work day for many of the surgical crew, as well as the anesthesiologist, pathologist and radiologist. All in order to please Dr. Haims.

Idly, Hank wondered what the surgical crew thought about having their Sundays free now. Were they happy with the rearranging of their personal schedules? Or did they miss the overtime pay, which they had gotten used to and had already spent, assuming it would always be there?

Corky caught his arm and drew him into conversation with a few friends. The talk was about funding the local art show sponsored by the college. She had been the mistress of ceremonies in its early beginnings. Like all pioneering endeavors, the first attempts were the most fun for everyone.

The discussion became quite animated and quite predictable. Artists were never appreciated in the smaller towns because their prices were barely affordable to the usual citizen, even though their adjusted prices were half that usually charged. It was a hard sell but no one was willing to give up trying.

A few voices, typically strained with appreciation, were leaving at the door. The evening had gone quickly.

Hank was pleased that nothing was said about his change in status in the hospital. Or about questions involving Dr. Haims's death. But then, they had avoided the difficult people and kept to their usual group of friends. It was time to leave. They were well on their way to the door when their luck ran out.

Thirteen

Dr. Span was suddenly standing in their path, antagonistic as always, but now the alcohol had eliminated what little governor there was on his usual thoughts.

"So, the incompetent pathologist is here!" he exclaimed with a smirk. His glassy eyes tried to focus in on them. They could hear sharp intakes of breath. The room fell silent.

"Misdiagnoses! Criminal malpractice! Laboratory error! What we need are some decent pathologists," Span continued. "How can anyone practice medicine with no backup at all? We're in the Dark Ages…the Middle Ages…as far as getting any help from the laboratory."

Span raised his arm for emphasis and the drink in his

glass flung into the air. "It isn't enough...enough that they kill patients but...they will autopsy anybody...dead or alive!"

The more he talked, the more he began to babble. Most of the listeners began walking away.

Seeing the loss of an audience, Span began to shout, swaying and spilling his drink. "And now, I'd better watch it or I'll get what Haims got." He made a motion of a gun being fired into his head. "And there's pathologist who can do it and leave no clues!" He pointed at Hank.

Hank pushed past him, towing Corky protectively with one arm, and went to the door.

"Cover up!" Span shouted. "Coverup! One pathologist kills you and another pathologist covers it up! It was Haims today, but tomorrow it'll be one of you! Ha! Ha!"

Darlene pushed through the crowd and appeared at the door. She looked stricken. "I'm sorry," she said.

Corky murmured something about not being able to control everything that happened at a party and graciously murmured their appreciation for the invitation.

Conversation at the party had now resumed as before. Span's shouting was now being ignored. Was it well known that with the loss of Haims, Span was reduced to the fill-in type of hospital committees—all work and no authority?

Span's wife finally appeared and grimly took him in hand. They disappeared into the crowd.

Hank and Corky left with dampened spirits. It didn't help that the evening had turned cold and threatened rain. The streets were deserted and the dark shadows fell and rose like ghosts along the sides of the car.

When would winter cease? Their winters were relatively mild but even so, the dark skies and rain were depressing.

Arriving home, they paid the baby sitter and Hank

drove her home. When Hank returned, Corky was still sitting on the edge of the bed, dressed and staring into space.

"Why is it always turmoil where you are?" she began. "Why can't things be pleasant and happy? Why couldn't you have gone into some other field? Are other doctors always criticized?"

Hank sat down heavily next to her. Every specialty had its problems. No field in medicine was without its critics— even research.

Being married to a physician was difficult at best and being married to a "hospital doctor," where it was open season on the laboratorians, appeared even worse. All labs performed over several thousand test analyses a day. The chances of error, even computer error, much less human error, were large. Add to that three shifts of employees, eighty-five in their practice, with part-timers covering the weekends. Running any twenty-four-hour operation was fraught with problems. The lab managed to capture its share. And also capture its share of irate physicians.

This week alone, one of their best technologists had performed ten pregnancy tests and reported them opposite to what they should have been. For some reason, the drug company had oriented the test so that a positive ring on the bottom of the test tube meant it was negative for pregnancy and the absence of a ring was positive for pregnancy. All the other chemical tests in the laboratory had positive reactions for positive tests.

As a result of the erroneous reporting, two people got married and the others had mixed reactions to their test results, which were even more mixed after they learned that the reverse was true. There were brief but very unhappy repercussions.

Hank put his arm around Corky and repeated what

must have been the same litany of words used throughout the ages by a husband to a wife. They had the good luck of having health, fine children, a nice roof over their heads and a job that was fulfilling.

He then began talking about a vacation in the mountains with the horses. This was Corky's most happy subject and Hank felt like a parent bringing up a toy bribe to appease a dejected child. But then, weren't they all children, playing grown-up games?

They went to bed eventually, not feeling better but at least having talked things out. The depressive mood still lingered with them the next morning at breakfast like a dark ogre waiting to engulf everything—home, children, all.

There had to be a turning point sometime.

Fourteen

At the roundup grounds, Corky looked up as she was tightening the cinch. Her horse had expanded her lungs and made it difficult to pull the straps tight.

"Dammit, Seaga!" she shouted. "Quit it."

A voice behind her interrupted her aggravation. "Why not walk her and tighten gradually?"

Without turning, Corky said, "Because she doesn't always bloat up with air—just now and then." Not recognizing the voice immediately, she looked over her shoulder at the speaker.

"Why Alex! What are you doing down here? Are you taking up the horse world?"

"Never will this wretched body place itself willingly in a vulnerable position on a walking trampoline. I came to see you."

"To see me? Why here?"

"Less formal. More relaxed environment."

"I'm interested." Corky frowned as her eyes were wary with surprise. She motioned to the children to ride off.

"Yes?" She began to walk with the horse, expecting Alex to follow when she realized he had a stumbling gait and stopped.

"I came to discuss your husband and his travails," he began.

"Now I'm really interested. Are you offering to help? Haims's death doesn't seem to have changed anything much for Hank."

Alex laughed. "You immediately plunge into the heart of a matter, don't you! I came to tell you that I've been empathizing, watching him silently agonize over his problems at the hospital. It must seem to him that he has no friends at all that are willing to come forward and be counted."

"That's for sure!" Corky answered. "Why doesn't he leave and get into something else? I've gotten so angry at him just doing nothing about all those put-downs! It isn't worth it to be attacked so persistently. It's like watching someone being eaten by ants."

"That's exactly why I came here to see you, Corky. This is only an observation, but a personal one. As I see it, this world has different kinds of heroes. He's the ordinary kind. No call for glory. No great expectations of recognition. He does his work, is proud of it, and he's good at it. You say he should leave? He's needed and that's his main satisfaction. The money isn't that great compared to other specialties, but the total commitment that the job requires is what attracts him. Is he that much different from all the other people in the country who just try to do their job, raise a family and get on with it?"

"No." Corky kicked the dirt with the toe of her boot. "But as his wife, I feel protective. He's taken so much garbage! I know he's not appreciated there! The administrator is urging him to leave by cutting his salary and position. The doctors feel it's not their ox that's being gored. And it's a rare patient that knows he even exists—much less that he often made the initial crucial diagnosis! I guess that's what galls me! Why stay where you're not appreciated?"

"Just the point I was attempting to make. Appreciation is not his way of thinking. He apparently is mature enough not to require the ego stroking that other doctors ordinarily receive. I'm rather envious of him, you know."

Alex looked embarrassed at the last statement, as though he had revealed a secret.

"Envious? Of Hank? Why? You both have the same training. You both perform the same work." Corky's mouth flew open.

"Ah, yes," said Alex. "Similar training. Homogenizing of knowledge. But unlike Hank, I refuse to hide my light under a bushel. I seek glory. Wantonly. I research and get published in the scientific community and then lard my conversations with these findings. I have a title of professor at the nearby college and mention that in any discourse. It's a form of puffery and I'm aware of it. Service to my fellow physicians, in the form of advice and diagnoses, earns my pay at St. Mary's. No more."

"My father says laboratory people are actually hiding from the real world. Is this true?" mused Corky.

"For me, it is! As for patients, I found that sick individuals were interesting to me only if they had a rare or unusual disease which I could study in depth and investigate. I don't enjoy my colleagues that much and freely admit it. On the other hand, I do enjoy being admired by them—or envied—no matter. But my point is, *my* thing wouldn't suit your husband at all! It's like the infantry soldier in the trenches and the officer sitting in Paris or Saigon. I am *not* the infantry soldier, by instinct, but I'm offering to become one—if Hank wants me!"

"You have an interesting outlook on life, Alex."

"To each his own, dear lady."

"Well, thanks for your time and for telling me this. It does help. You make a good friend, Alex."

"No, Corky. Sadly, I wish I did. At the first sign of rancor or combat, I desist and retreat. Unlike your husband, I feel no compunction to draw a battle line...'this far you may go and no farther.' Alex Trueheart, I am not."

"Then why did you take the time to come down here and explain all this about Hank?" asked Corky.

"Self-interest. Hank's type often prevails, just as faith, truth, wisdom, genuineness has prevailed over the centuries. He is a far more complex personality than either you or I give him credit for, you know. I'd like to stay in the laboratory in the same position. Under Hank, I would. Under Schmidt...well...the Schmidts of the world are successful, sometimes enormously successful—but only for a short time. They self-destruct, so to speak."

Corky pulled on the cinch. As she did so, her horse showed her displeasure by flattening her ears. "You're full of puzzling *observations*, Alex. You say Hank is a complex personality? I'm his wife. I know him well. I've born his babies and have been with him for years. You only see him in the hospital."

"Ah, yes. Adversity brings out certain hidden character traits that you wouldn't know existed—even in your best of friends—much less your husband. In some, it only reveals the flaws. I merely wish to admonish you not to be surprised at a change in his personality."

"Whew! Am I to expect the growth of horns and sharp teeth? Should I make a daily check of this forehead and jaw?" laughed Corky.

Alex's eyes flickered. "I'm only discharging a self-imposed obligation by expressing a few perceptions about your husband and his present position. Please accept them as such. When the time comes and he'd like to open an independent shop, I would like to be considered a partner."

"I'm sorry. I really appreciate the time you have taken and I didn't mean to ridicule what you said. Hank is such a good man and to have him..." Corky put her boot in the stirrup and swung up easily. "He'll decide about leaving on his own, you know."

"Over time, good men prevail, Corky. That could be an aphorism, couldn't it? Sloppy and saccharine."

Corky smiled. "Embarrassed at sentiment, are you?" she said. "Well, thanks again for being a friend and offering to join him. I won't forget...and neither will Hank."

Alex smiled, bowed slightly and as he left in his stumbling gait, the vision of the smiling rider up against the sky remained with him for several moments and almost made him want to ride as well. But...no, never that. He shook his head vigorously. Just the same, a hint of a smile began to form on his lips and he began to whistle.

Indeed, it was a beautiful day. A day to be enjoyed. Hopefully, he had done the right thing. Since it made him feel so good, he probably had!

Fifteen

When Hank came into the laboratory Monday, the secretary notified him that Dr. Schmidt wanted to see him right away. Hank went into his former office.

Schmidt was sitting at the desk writing. He looked comfortable in a new chair. The room was changed and all Hank's pictures were replaced with Schmidt's diplomas. It was impressive. Hank reflected he had as many and more but kept them in a drawer at home. Sometimes, he pulled them out and stared at the fancy writing and emblems as though they belonged to someone else.

"You wanted to see me?"

"Yes," Schmidt said. He looked up briefly and continued to write. "The police think you are involved with Dr. Haims's murder."

"I know." Hank felt a dull thud land in his groin. Now that the news was circulating, what ploy was Schmidt going to use?

"You're definitely being investigated. Questions are being asked." Schmidt looked flustered as he always did when he spoke to Hank. "It's hurting the lab."

"How?"

"Well, we've got our professional reputation to maintain and your involvement as a suspect injures us all. We've got to do something to assure the doctors that we're reliable!"

"And?" Hank wasn't going to make it easier for him.

"Well..." Schmidt looked even more agitated. "Perhaps you could think of something."

"I can't. Schmidt, you're trying every way you can to push me out. I'm not going."

"Well, you do agree it looks bad for the lab to have someone around who is a suspect in a murder?"

"No, I can't see why they suspect me, but it's self-serving on your part to suggest that I'm involved."

Their eyes locked and Schmidt's frustration flared up in his eyes and his mustache almost formed a circle. "In that case, there is nothing to talk about." Schmidt imperially dismissed Hank by picking up his writing material and reading it.

"Right...Your Majesty." Hank grimaced. Who said the meek inherit the earth?

It was obvious that Schmidt, true or not, was going to insert the subject of his being a suspect in all hospital conversations.

Hank had to do something or his job would be gone. Who were the other suspects? The police would have the raw data.

He couldn't check all this unless he took off some time. Who would cover for him? Not Ed or Schmidt. That left Alex. How could he ask Alex, the observer of life, who avoided any real contact with people?

Alex had said some kind things to him and went out of his way to contact Corky about his situation on Saturday. A strange man. Well read. Honors in literature. Master's in English. That alone, majoring in literature and still obtaining the necessary chemistry and physics for medicine, made him different. Medical schools said they wanted their students "well-rounded," but everyone knew they only looked at your grades in the sciences and often solely at the numbers on the national medical aptitude test. Hank wondered what had happened to Alex in his life that made him so aloof and obsessed with his privacy. Still, he would make a capable and honest partner if it came to that.

Hank went to his back office, cleared up a few pending cases that had to be finalized and called the police chief's department for an appointment. Shortly after, the secretary called back and confirmed a 9:30 A.M. time. Interestingly, this was the time they usually met at the Bolli.

"Coffee?" The trustee at the police station was a toothless, freshly shaven, old-time inebriate who waved a pot of coffee at him. He was clad in green army-type fatigues and he obviously reveled in his role of serving the police. Hank wondered if he also didn't secretly enjoy entertaining thoughts of poisoning the whole staff.

"Yes. Thanks."

The trustee poured the coffee into a ceramic mug.

"No plastic cups?"

"No, sir! No plastic! We're high-class people around here. Chief's orders!" The trustee grinned, showing his missing teeth.

Detective Monty was in the room with chief Enzer.

"Dr. Haims's murder," Hank decided to state the problem clearly. "Apparently, the hospital is buzzing with talk that I'm being investigated and am a suspect."

They both looked at the desktop and then stared at Hank without speaking. His problem was his problem. They weren't going to help at all. Hank could see it was time to stop using a slingshot.

"I've worked with you and your department for over ten years. We've solved some difficult cases together. Now I need to know something. You suspect me of murder. You've must have all kinds of information—don't tell me it's classified—I know it's classified. But I need to know some of it, even if it's only to refute the implications."

They shifted their eyes and looked at each other. Silence. The chief spoke first. "In any murder investigation, everyone with a motive who could have been at the scene…" Hank nodded impatiently and waited. "…and you had a motive."

Hank said nothing. It was useless. All policemen and lawyers tended not to believe what a suspect says. It was infuriating to those who were truthful and a role reversal for Hank. But at least he was intellectually aware of their thoughts, even if emotionally it was hard.

He could have been at the scene of the crime. "You said motive?" he questioned.

"Yes."

"Who else had a motive?"

"A number."

"I hope some had a stronger motive than mine?"

"Perhaps." The chief almost lost his studied poker face.

"Who did you check out?"

"Wife, rest of family, friends, other colleagues, patients…" Monty and the chief took turns replying blandly.

First one, then the other. Almost disinterestedly.

"Remember the case that I recommended for DNA fingerprinting? How did that come out?" Hank asked.

Both men shifted position. That case involved a drop of blood left on the doorjamb at the stabbing scene. They were going to get the usual blood tests and weren't aware of the genetic research just available that could pinpoint the exact person who perpetrated the crime. The DNA analysis solved the crime and they had been very appreciative...then.

Hank continued reciting case after case in which they had worked together. The type of weapon used by assailant after assailant he had reconstructed, judging from the pattern of the skull fractures or wounds. They began to shift uneasily and finally looked at each other.

"You're boxing us in," said Chief Enzer.

"Had to...you're both acting like asses suspecting me of murder!" said Hank.

Monty wiped both of his hands together, looked at the chief who nodded, and then opened his hands outwardly, defensively.

"Okay. We'll chance it. At first, there appeared to be little to go on. The insurance to his wife was no motive, since he would have earned more alive than dead. No known evidence of marital discord. No girlfriends found so far. A search of the room yielded nothing...no letters, no incriminating evidence. Outside the grounds...nothing. Windows...no tampering. No footprints, but it was a dry, rainless week. Neighbors heard nothing. The only real fact we have is that he was shot in the head with his own gun and his wife stated she avoided anything to do with his gun collection."

"But he had an enemy or enemies who wanted him dead," said Hank.

Monty pointedly answered, "We figured you would know about that better than us. We gave you a chance to detail us about your arguments with him and you didn't."

Hank looked at them grimly. "Internal hospital stuff."

"Not to us," the chief spoke, half-explaining and half-justifying his actions. "You were a suspect because of your fight with Haims and things he had said about you. Yep. Don't look surprised. It was reported ten different ways. He was going to get you out of St. Mary's. When you couldn't verify your whereabouts at the time of Dr. Haims's death and when the perpetrator left no clue…well, we have to consider all possibilities—even though you have been our pathologist."

"Of course," Hank agreed. "You're up against someone who knew how to kill and plan it well. One bullet. Right spot. Quick, clean kill. Immediate death. How to manage a gunshot sound so it would remain unreported—only a professional would know."

Both men nodded at Hank's summary.

"But you two forgot something. There was a blow to the back of the head. And some other things. What about them?"

The chief got up and walked around the desk. Hank knew the chief well enough to know he was angry even though he didn't seem to change expression. "At the scene, I saw you check for rigor mortis and examine the bloody area on the back of the head. Dr. Schmidt said the skull fracture could have been caused by the force of the bullet bouncing around the inside of the skull," he said.

"That type of skull fracture? Christ!" The words spilled out of Hank.

"What?" Monty's and the chief's heads snapped up.

"Yes."

"Tell us more." Both men were became fully alert, then wary.

"It's not my autopsy. Schmidt wouldn't let me see his final protocol—I only observed a few things at the scene and in the morgue."

"There *was* a skull fracture due to the bullet," Chief Enzer offered, trying to draw Hank out.

Hank shook his head. "I'll tell you more when you let me see some of your investigative files. A trade. No files, no discussion."

Reluctantly, the chief picked up the phone and spoke. A few moments later, an officer brought in a thick file. The chief flipped through the file, picked out some papers and kept them. The remainder he shoved over to Hank.

"How much time do I have?" Hank asked.

"We'll tell you. Go ahead."

Hank began to read as fast as he could and took notes. It was no use asking to use their copy machine.

St. Mary's Hospital records for staff membership were there. He started with these. It was odd to see his application in his handwriting together with that of Haims's. Haims had begun his practice in Texas. This lasted for about two years. He moved to Michigan, where he practiced for three years. Then he moved to a small town in upper Washington State for two years. This was actually the fourth move because he came to Red Wolf by way of Seattle, where he worked for less than a year.

Unexplained gaps were there, which should have been red flags to any credential's committee. The move to Michigan from Texas was explainable. A second move so quickly became suspect. A third move in such a short time is always questioned by a credentials committee. But then, a move to a small town, and then to a large city, Seattle. And then to Red Wolf? What about the large gaps of time in between?

The credentials committee at St. Mary's had sloughed

their homework. Was it because they needed a general surgeon so badly that any warm, licensed body would do? A few phone calls to the right people would have given them the necessary information. Schizoid personalities were all too often successful in every field. Intelligence was not impaired. Only interaction with others. Alternately warm and solicitous, then angry and demanding, then abject apologies followed by sympathetic interest, then sudden hatred and annihilation of anyone vulnerable. Schizoid. An apt name for those with one foot in reality and one foot in paranoia.

Unanswered questions. Like the need to cheat when Haims already earned much more than the average physician. Once earned, where did it go? Secret investments? Was money a motive for the killing? Money, the powerful aphrodisiac. Why did it claim such importance in someone professing strong religious beliefs? Unless he was funding something for the church.

Sam Sager, Haims's partner, was there. So was Keith Gray. Surprise! What was Keith doing in the file? Span was included. Cliff Evers had been interviewed. Mrs. Haims had been reinterviewed—it seemed to be regarding one of the children who had been on hard drugs and was in and out of institutions. Drugs meant money and money meant stealing. Was this Haims's problem, his child needing expensive rehabilitation? But Haims had injured someone enough to make that person want to kill him. Who?

Investigators always started with someone close to the person. Family. Friends. Coworkers. First question: Who would benefit?

Hank Whipple would benefit. With Haims gone, his job would be secure—Span wouldn't have any power in committees—and all his problems should be solved eventually.

Smooth job. No clues. You bet he himself would place Hank Whipple amongst the suspects, if he were investigating!

His thoughts were interrupted. "Tell us what you know about the death of Haims." Impatient eyes stared at him.

"Show me the protocol and the photographs and I'll point out what I saw," said Hank.

Another file was brought in. It contained raw data about the scene of the crime, photos of the scene and Schmidt's autopsy report.

Hank pointed to what he considered of paramount importance in the photographs. Quickly, he skimmed the autopsy report and stated his opinions about several aspects, summarizing what was missing. Under the circumstances, he felt he owed Schmidt no loyalty. He looked up.

The eyes that looked back at him were not appreciative of the new knowledge—on the contrary—they were cloudy with suspicion.

Startled, Hank realized that if he had been just one of many suspects before, then his explanations only served to make him an even stronger suspect now.

He was in it deeper than ever. Now he'd better do something and fast!

Sixteen

When Hank returned to the hospital from the police station, an autopsy authorization had been signed by the family of the deceased. Several phone numbers were listed on the face sheet of different attending physicians. When many physicians wish to be called on the autopsy results, it meant one thing: that particular autopsy was going to cause someone an amount of unhappiness.

But that was the pathologist's job—an independent, unbiased opinion. He read the chart. Male. Seventy-two years old. Found dead next to toilet on floor. Multiple illnesses.

He announced the beginning time of the autopsy on

the hospital paging system by saying, "CPC for doctors and nurses in the laboratory." CPC stood for clinical pathological conference.

The morgue presented the usual setting. Predictable almost every time. The morgue table was partly surrounded by five nurses-to-be. Four female and one male. All were jostling with each other for the back of the group and yet trying to appear blase. The two in front were avoiding the staring eyes of the corpse.

"First time for all of you?" The answer was a vigorous nodding. Half-embarrassed smiles. They had been coerced into coming to the morgue since it was part of their training requirements.

Hank Whipple began his preliminary talk with a mental sigh. Once again, he had to wipe out preconceived ideas of ghouls, evil spirits, Dracula and any recent terror movies about violence. If they only knew how he personally avoided viewing any bloodletting on television. What would they think if they knew Walt Disney was a hero of his? An escapist?

He took photographs from every angle of the body. This was not usual in hospital cases but necessary when sticky situations arose. During the photography, he attempted to explain the procedure to be performed was similar to any surgical operation.

The words were almost a litany. "The body is examined just as you would a living, human being. We're here to ascertain the cause of death. This involves reviewing the chart and correlating the signs and symptoms with the treatment given. Another purpose of the autopsy is to find any disease or significant entity missed in the original diagnosis or to find any communicable disease that would involve the family or hospital personnel in contact with the patient.

"Since no two people are alike, no two autopsies will be alike. It's important to follow a fairly rigid protocol in our examination. That way, nothing will be missed.

"First, we begin by observation, without touching the body. Head. Trunk. Extremities. General condition of the person—appear older or younger than the stated age of seventy-two years? Shaved, unshaved? Fingernails trimmed, untrimmed, polish? Hair rinsed, colored? Any marks, scars? Anything out of the ordinary? Position of body? Rigor mortis? Livor mortis? What do those words mean?"

He looked up. The students were shrinking away and avoiding eye contact. Wrong tact. Ask and answer was always best when you're not sure of their knowledge level at school. The intimidation method of the Germanic school of medical teaching he had undergone was wrong. People only remembered being intimidated. So he asked and answered his own questions.

"Rigor mortis is a coagulation of muscle tissue much like the colorless white of an egg changes into something visible and white—only rigor mortis disappears in twenty-four to forty-eight hours. Its appearance usually begins at the face, noted easiest with the masseter muscles, and continues downward, ending at the extremities. It disappears in the order it appeared. The time of appearance and disappearance are dependent upon the size of the body, fever or its absence, and the general physical condition prior to demise.

"In the present patient, rigor mortis is well-developed throughout the entire body. Do you agree?"

One student voiced: "But he's in the sitting position."

"True. Note that both arms are floppy, yet the remainder of the body is unyielding. Why? I just got through stating the path of beginning and lessening of the rigor, yet the arms are loose…" The students were quiet. He waited and then answered his own question. "Someone manipulated the arms and broke the rigor—probably to make transporting the body easier through the hospital wards. Agreed?

"Livor mortis is the settling of blood into the dependent portions of the body—caused by the force of gravity. This is rarely considered important in hospital deaths, since almost everyone dies in bed and the blood settles into the posterior half or back part of the body. In forensic work, this finding can be a very important factor. Here we note the deep-red color beginning in the lower trunk and involving both lower legs. Compare this with the color of the head, upper trunk and upper extremities. Is there a difference?"

They nodded and the same student asked: "This would mean the patient died in a sitting position, then."

"True. But the doctor's orders in this chart state that the patient must be assisted to the bathroom. What happened?"

The nurses looked at each other. One replied, "He went without asking for help...and died."

They were on the right track. The patient was found partly sprawled on the floor next to the commode, hours after he had died. Too many hours.

"Perhaps. How would you explain the rigor mortis then, if he was declared dead forty minutes ago? He's not excessively thin, not debilitated and did not have a high fever. Rigor mortis would be expected to begin in six to eight hours, and yet rigor is well-advanced..."

The nurses now looked sideways at each other. Something unpleasant was coming up.

"Hint. When was the patient checked last?"

The students huddled over the chart. The one student began to serve as a spokesperson: "Notes are written that he was satisfactory right up to half an hour before he was discovered dead."

He looked at the students steadily. "Also TPRs—temperature, pulse and respirations—are carefully recorded right up to the end, aren't they?"

They all read the temperature, pulse, respiration chart carefully. Puzzled, they looked up.

"Does it add up?"

Again, they looked at each other without speaking. Someone had done the unthinkable. The TPRs had been falsely written down, probably ahead of time. Now the recording nurse was caught, right down to her initials at the bottom of each written notation.

The embarrassment passed. The rest of the autopsy went easily. The patient was elderly and had multiple problems. The heart exhibited advanced hardening of the arteries. Hank took the usual representative samples from each organ and placed the tissues in a bottle of preserving buffered formalin.

"Approximately two centimeters from the origin of the coronary ostia, hard yellow material partly closes the opening so that only 20 percent is left for the blood to flow through and nourish the heart. The right coronary vessel is 50 percent occluded. What is one of the causes of arteriosclerosis?"

This was easy and less threatening. They soon became engrossed in a discussion about food, cholesterol, heredity and exercise. The familiar question of the value of exercise was raised. "Could he have reversed the 'rusty pipes' with exercise?"

"Probably not at the age of seventy-two," Hank said. "The best he could hope for is developing collateral circulation. At a younger age, it's probable, and depends upon each individual. A few years ago, a cardiologist stated he had never noted a cardiac death in a marathon runner. Shortly after this statement, a marathon runner died a cardiac death. Then another died while jogging. Of course, there's the story of Jim Fixx..." The rest of the post-mortem exam went at a comfortable pace and as the students relaxed, they began arguing among themselves about various organs, their functions and how you could tell whether or not they were normal. Their minds forgot the dripping blood from gloved hands holding various organs, the sweet, musty smell of the opened body cavity and the continuous sound of running water.

Hank felt a wave of satisfaction. The students had forgotten their antipathy to a dead body and now were engrossed in the findings.

This was the satisfying part of an autopsy—transferring the excitement of learning. It was learning at its best. Not dull anatomy and pictures in books to memorize. Not dull lectures and colored slides. But examining real tissue that presented the disease or malfunction leading to death. How to prevent it—how to help the condition once it had taken hold of a person—what to do—what not to do. What not to do. That indeed. *Primum non nocere*—First do no harm.

Hank's exuberance fell when he thought of his report. The hospital authorities would have mixed feelings about the results. He would have to return the doctor's calls and give them his findings. They would be angry and file incident reports. Nursing service was faced with an immediate problem: a nurse was faking vital signs. The autopsy would document it and now the hospital's legal department would worry about a lawsuit. He could see the documents now: "The pathologist has found..."

Faking results was an ever-present concern in all facets of patient care—including his own laboratory techs. It was a little like embezzling. It first began with small things that supposedly didn't matter—at least they told themselves it didn't matter—and then, when not caught out, the acts progressively escalated.

Hank sewed up the body quickly. While washing up prior to leaving, he overheard students conversing and saying, "It wasn't anything like I thought it was going to be!" The students left.

He hadn't told them about the repercussions from the doctors and administration. Doctors and hospitals had mixed feelings about autopsy authorizations and requesting them. The poorer the doctor, the less likely he wanted an autopsy.

Returning to his office, he dictated his findings and set the tissues in small plastic cassettes for the histologist to process into slides. The film he sent with the courier to be developed.

A thick envelope of letters was on his desk. All had been faxed. It was from the Seattle group of pathologists. Did they confirm or disagree with his diagnoses?

His heart suddenly pounding, he began leafing through the consultation reports. It was like being graded in school again. There was a tremble in his hands as his eyes sought the final diagnoses at the bottom of each page.

They shone like written gold:

Agree with diagnosis.
Agree with diagnosis.
Agree with diagnosis.

There had been nothing wrong with his diagnoses! Where was the criminal aspect? Who reviewed his slides for Dr. Span?

Hank picked up the phone angrily, then realized it was

the wrong time to converse with Dr. Span. Once again, Dr. Span was not available. At least now, Hank knew Span was lying.

He took the faxed reports and copied them. Placing each on the pathologists' desks, he wrote: "You needn't check my diagnoses anymore!" Next, he sent copies to each of the members of the ad hoc committee and to the administrator of St. Mary's.

He felt lightheaded with the pleasure of having his diagnoses corroborated—but the pleasure was short-lived. Nothing had really changed that much. He was still a prime murder suspect. A much stronger suspect—now that he had pointed out the probable sequence of events in the photos and missing material in the autopsy.

What was he going to do about it? Waiting was foolish. He had read enough of the police files to know whom they had contacted and the direction of their investigation. He had better start clearing himself.

Seventeen

Corky rang. "Remember I told you that the children and I were going home to Wisconsin for a week?"

Yes, he had remembered but repressed it. "Are you leaving now?"

"Yes. I told you this morning." Corky expected him to mentally block their leaving. She discussed the things he should do to keep up the house and the chores at the Roundup Grounds.

"My diagnoses were correct, according to the Seattle pathologists," Hank heard himself say rather proudly.

"I thought they would be," replied Corky. "You take these vindictive games too seriously. I'm glad you're relieved, but there was no doubt in my mind. Goodbye!"

On the drive home, the road curved along the Clearwater River, surrounded by the many pine trees, colorful bushes and high rolling hills. Spring covered the hills with early pale-green buds in patches, so that there was a strong contrast with the brown and green of the wet soil and rocks.

He was reminiscing how friendships were like chemical compounds, made up of hundreds upon hundreds of molecules, but only certain ones attracted each other and remained firmly bound; others clung momentarily but easily became dislodged, and still others repelled and would never combine, even under the most drastic conditions.

A warm, steady bond was not present with his own colleagues in the pathology department? Sadly, each doctor went his own way. Consulting between them was usually formal, analytical, and even the disagreements were perfunctory and automatically sent for outside consultant's opinions.

Wasn't this his fault as the director? No. The men were not of his choosing. They were hired and paid by the hospital; since their credentials were satisfactory, acceptable to all.

Perhaps part of the problem in practicing pathology was that the patient was not personally known or even seen, so the aches and pains of the patient were unperceived and the patient became a case. But when you knew the person, like Cliff Evers, and realized his suffering—well, that became different.

In some ways, it was better not to know the individual because it kept objectivity as a primary focus but the warmth of human relationships was lost and the enjoyment of the art of medicine, that essential part of practice ignored by third-party insurers, was not to be part of the practice of pathology.

Were all scholarly endeavors thus so? Yes, even back in the days of Pasteur. Thinkers were lonely doves that always preferred the isolated atmosphere and flew together all too briefly. The lack of camaraderie in the laboratory wasn't his fault as director. Any major achievements or break-throughs were lonely ones, thought out alone, and final-ized after many long hours of winding through the mul-tiple blind experimental mazes, each requiring decision and discipline.

Busy in his thoughts, Hank suddenly found his car spinning toward the other side of the road, heading for the large outcropping of rock. His reflexes caused him to overcorrect and the car circled into a scary spin, circling once, and then twice, until Hank remembered to turn the car wheels opposite to the spin and on the third go-around, the car went into the gravel on the other side of the road, facing the direction he was coming from.

The side of the car landed at the edge of the road just above the Clearwater River. After the first spin, he had unlocked the seatbelt, expecting the car to roll into the water, only to find the car making still another circle.

The ground was wet. He got out and went back, looking at the road for an oil slick or for ice. His heart was now pounding with adrenalin.

There was nothing—just ordinary, wet pavement. It was his own fault. He had been speeding home on a wet, rain-swept road while concentrating on his problems.

Was this an omen? A sign telling him to stop being so preoccupied with himself and to get on what he had to do? Strange how he believed in signs like these. A scientist believing in omens. How amusing it would be to others if he tried to explain his belief in such omens.

Hank had waited passively for someone to come to his

defense. If he wasn't forced out by Schmidt, his place in the laboratory would be a satellite role. When Haims's murder was solved, shouldn't he just change hospitals? Start again? Was it worth it to stay on at St. Mary's in this situation?

The answer was yes. The work was important, satisfying and he knew he was good at it. Now he could prove his diagnoses were satisfactory.

The omen with the vehicle he felt was portentous and he resolved to forget everything and immerse himself in work. There were improvements to be made in the laboratory. For one, the immunochemistry stains needed upgrading. The new peroxidase techniques were in the forefront, but the reagents were a concern.

Too many companies were in the marketplace too early, without a single one waiting to manufacture a quality product with sufficient sensitivity and specificity. Market share was everything today.

When he entered the immuno-chemistry section, Steve Blodgett, the salesman for one of the less reliable companies, was there talking to the techs. Blodgett seemed ebullient. Hank wondered why?

Digger, the supervisory tech, called over and said, "You met Steve Blodgett of Hempter Laboratories?" Hank nodded. Digger's face was noncommittal as he said, "He tells me he just got an exclusive five-year contract to supply us with Hempter's reagents."

For Digger to act noncommittal was akin to rejection, but Blodgett was too ecstatic to notice. He kept turning on his charm in all directions of the room.

Hank felt himself burning. Lab supplies shouldn't be ordered without input from a pathologist. Hempter's reagents were unsatisfactory.

He heard himself say, "Who did you bribe, Blodgett? Hempter has the worst reputation for reliability in the market." It was an abrasive approach. Uncouth, but then, so was the salesman.

Blodgett's face reflected several quick changes as he looked at Hank with surprise. His eyes bulged with the effort of first denial, then bluster, and finally, Blodgett decided to register shock at the direct insult.

Digger's face broke into a bright smile and he could hardly hold back the quick laugh as he listened for the answer.

"Dr. Whipple," said Blodgett, "we only deal with those in authority. You're no longer in charge here. People who really know, respect our reputation for quality. Our re-agents have been used by—"

"You have no quality, as far as I'm concerned. You shouldn't even be allowed to market your products, they're so unreliable," Hank continued angrily.

"Then I'm glad someone in authority thinks differently. I have a five-year contract!" said Blodgett meaningfully.

"It's a payoff, Blodgett. You know it and I know it."

Blodgett looked around the room and saw that all the other bench techs had stopped working and were quietly listening.

"That's insulting!" he said. "I don't have to listen to this garbage from you. You just take orders!" He got up and left the laboratory.

Digger looked up and smiled wanly. "That wasn't very nice of you—after all, he brought us all two big boxes of donuts and pastries."

Blodgett was right, though. Hank did "just take orders," as he said. It did not leave a good feeling, but this had not been their first clash about Hempter's products.

Hempter Laboratories was a large conglomerate, well-known in the trade to spare no expense in subsidizing general medical meetings and lavish parties. Hospitals thought kindly of Hempter because of their generous donations to any cause the hospital deemed important or necessary.

Hempter also promoted hospital and medical seminars in enchanting foreign countries and picked up all the bills, including travel costs. It was well-known and even tacitly accepted in medical circles, that anyone showing interest in Hempter's products would be automatically invited to their special seminars and incidentally, presented with gifts commensurate with the person's prestige, committee chairmanship and quantity of product usage.

But the tar brush painted broadly because other medical supply companies did the same thing for years but were less obvious. Hempter made no attempt to disguise it for what it was—quid pro quo—merely a business expense in order to get more business. One had to admire their honesty, if not their promotion methods.

"Where are the Hempter reagents, Digger?

"In the refrigerator next to the first post on the right."

Hank went over and pulled out the chemicals, carried them to the waste basket and threw them in. Everyone was watching. He heard someone say, "That's all they're good for." But he didn't bother to look up.

"What'll we do when we get orders for those tests?" asked Digger hesitantly.

"Send them out until we can get reagents from Ortho or Abbott, or someone we know is dependable."

Digger nodded unhappily now. It was his nature to keep things pleasant and now he knew trouble was coming. Like others, he tried to keep clear of controversy.

It was shortly after lunch that Carol Gardon, the lab secretary, called and told Hank that Dr. Schmidt wanted to see him.

"I'm right here, Carol, on the laboratory bench. I'm sure he can walk thirty steps."

About fifteen minutes later, a visibly annoyed Schmidt came into the lab. "Doctor, did you throw out hundreds of dollars of chemical reagents just now?"

Digger had reported the event and disappeared.

"Yes. They were worthless."

"Were they outdated or what? We can get credit for that."

"They were worthless, from a worthless company."

"The FDA approved them."

"On a research basis. They're still worthless."

"The hospital cannot afford throwing out expensive chemicals just on a whim. All the hospitals in this Order have contracted with Hempter chemicals and are satisfied."

"The blessing of the Hospital Order still doesn't make them decent chemicals."

"Either you take those chemicals out of the waste container or I'll have to report your actions to the hospital authorities. The choice is yours!"

They stared at each other. Schmidt already knew the reagents would remain discarded. Schmidt spun on his heel and left.

Bad vibrations continued to reverberate in the spot where he stood. The lab became dead quiet and only the hum of the computerized blood analyzers could be heard. The summons from administration wasn't long in coming.

Eighteen

Carol came into the lab and slipped him a note. Her face was wary. "Tim Hawkes asks that you see him at your earliest convenience."

Now was as good as ever. He left on the white coat; perhaps it might be good for some subtle psychological benefits.

Upstairs, Tim Hawkes was sitting with one hand under his chin and his elbow on the desk. He remained in this slumped-over position even after Hank entered and sat down.

How different it was a short time ago when they relaxed and laughed at their witticisms concerning the foibles of various members of the hospital staff. Tim's problems between doctors-nurses-patients-employees had a continuous flow to them.

Tim didn't speak but looked at Hank wordlessly.

"Trouble?" Hank asked.

"Yes." Tim stirred.

"Again?" A poor attempt at humor.

He only blinked. "Yes." There was no smile—no expression.

"The autopsy report—I couldn't do anything but report what I found."

Tim closed his eyes as though they were tired. "That's not an issue."

"I checked on the different cases which I diagnosed. They're all right! The ad hoc committee is mud-slinging..."

"Not an issue." Tim raised his eyebrows, as though commanding them would make everything unpleasant vanish.

Hank twisted in his chair. "Okay. It *is* about the reagents, then. They're not always accurate. One batch will be fine and the next will not. Our test results will not be dependable."

Tim sighed, sat up straight and took a moment to reflect and then speak. "I understand your point. I'm not a doctor. I can't tell you what to do. I can only tell you that, as a cost-cutting measure, the mother hospital in Minnesota contracts for supplies in the name of all the hospitals in their Order. They are adamant about saving on all hospital supplies, including laboratory supplies. It works. They get the best advice, cost account everything, and make a decision. We abide by their decisions. They have been so successful, even non-Catholic hospitals have asked to join them and also save. It works."

"Hempter products don't always work."

"Dr. Schmidt says they do."

"He doesn't do the bench work. The techs will tell you."

"I've talked to them."

"Then you know."

Tim hesitated a moment and then said, "They say they can work with them."

"Because Dr. Schmidt got to them first." Hank realized he had just said the wrong thing. A child could have handled his pique better. And worded it better.

"I don't know that that is true." Tim's face was impassive. "It is expected that you would be resentful toward Dr. Schmidt under the circumstances, but I assure you I have never heard Dr. Schmidt speak of you except in the most respectful terms."

Tim's face was a quiet study. Not unfriendly, but on the other hand, cool, unemotional and definite. Just as you would when dealing with a recalcitrant child.

"Which means I have a choice."

"Yes." The voice of authority was speaking to a child.

Hank got up. Of course he could go to the mother house in Minnesota and state his case. But who would listen to a single voice objecting to the decisions carefully made by a group of full-time financial planners? Accounting experts were now the foundation of the hospitals. Without their interpretations of the latest rules of compensation from the governmental agencies and insurance companies, the hospitals would flounder and fail.

Like a foreign country, when you went into a territory, you either abided by the rules of that territory or you left. An academic degree or M.D. conferred no special immunity against flaunting the rules. Hank had voluntarily chosen the hospital territory to work in. Exceptions were not feasible.

That left no choice for the Rule-Enforcer. And no real choice for the Rule-Breaker.

Outside, the sunny sky was cloudy and a slight drizzle of rain misted over him as he walked to the car. Winter was coming. The omen on the drizzly road had come true. But it was due to his own rigid behavior. Or had he been set up for the entire episode by someone who knew how he would react?

Deep in his thoughts, he wasn't aware of a dark figure crowding him from one side of his car until he was tripped and found himself falling and struggling to stay up. The man was heavier than his form appeared. He jabbed a hard fist into Hank's face.

Still off-balance, Hank tried to catch the man's clothes and stay up and at the same time tried to fling him onto the car. He was unsuccessful. Two fists pounded on Hank's chest and left him breathless. The face above the fists was dark and showed intent, narrow eyes. Although shorter, the man was more muscular in every way.

Hank was losing the fight, which made him angry, but his anger did not make him more effective. It was not just a robbery he was up against, but hatred and hostility. Money was not demanded.

Headlights blazed, lit them up and moved rapidly at them. A screech of the tires and a large figure leaped out, yelling, "Hey! What's going on here?!"

The dark figure hid his face, punched once more, then fled, leaving Hank breathless and too weak to give chase. He squinted with relief at the new arrival.

"Thanks for coming by," Hank said breathlessly.

"You all right? What was that all about?" It was Sam Sager. Once again, Sam was backing him out of a tough spot.

"I don't know. The guy had a lot of ill will stored up."

Sam reached into his car and dialed. "You'll need to tell the police about it. It's probably a mugger working the hospital parking lot and you just happened to turn up."

Hank nodded but without conviction. Muggers demanded things. This one was intent on hurting.

Within five minutes, the police were there and asked the usual description questions. There wasn't much to tell. Chunky build, solid arms which he had felt during the grasping, about five foot ten, curly long hair, dressed in black. He couldn't remember any colors. The attack was wordless on both sides.

That was all. Except for the hatred.

"Who?" they asked and he had a strong suspicion.

After expressing his gratitude to Sam Sager, he refused going to the Emergency Room and went home to a quiet house.

Lonely and depressed. He hadn't noticed before how important noises were in the home. He had always accepted noise, happy noise, and now there was only the hum of the refrigerator.

Now he had another problem. Someone hated him but not enough to kill him. Just a good thrashing with perhaps a broken limb for remembrance.

Nineteen

He called Corky in Wisconsin but only her parents were available to talk and their conversation was all too brief. The generation gap manifested itself quickly because the expense of the long-distance call bothered them. It seemed Corky had hardly arrived when she left to visit childhood friends.

He called the hospital switchboard and had them forward all telephone calls to his home number and answering service.

Since he had another empty evening, he decided to check out all the possible suspects. Whom did he know in the various cities that would tell him the true facts? Fellow pathologists: they knew everything. He began calling.

The first call was a dud. So was the second. The third and fourth were very informative. He was finding out some important hidden facts about individuals. Hank exulted at the thought of what a small world it was in medicine.

Now he had some definite direction about the killing of Haims. Being a suspect was grating. It'd be a major relief to resolve this. His job came to mind. Or future job.

Actually there were many options. Research, teaching, direct patient care or continuing on in laboratory service as a pathologist. Those were just a few. Of course, there was always the option to leave medicine. But that was unthinkable.

The practice of medicine, in spite of all its problems, was the most marvelous privilege allowed any human being. With that thought, Hank realized for the first time, how locked-in he was, mentally.

No other useful or worthwhile work in life? Preposterous! What an arrogant thought! There was more to life than just the niche of practicing medicine!

There it was, though. It took adversity for him to admit that enjoyment of his work in medicine was akin to enjoyment of life. How did he get this mindset?

Regardless, he had to make some decisions immediately. Research would require funding and equipment—time-intensive factors which required long waits without assurance the specific research project would even be approved.

Teaching was generally done gratis by all physicians—rarely did one get an honorarium and Hank did need money to support his family. Universities? They were glad to have you donate your time and offered a clinical title, but it wasn't the same as a paying job.

Directing a private laboratory for a large group of

physicians was a possibility but most medical groups had to consider the bottom line as extremely important. The service aspects were paramount and any interesting side research would have to be out of his own pocket.

Giving up pathology and practicing direct patient care meant opening an office and slowly building up patients and their trust. Right now, there were enough physicians in town and they were scrambling for patients. At this time, he would be accepted but not really welcomed.

A private laboratory would thrive only if it were located conveniently near the doctors' offices. There was a small, empty building across the street from the hospital—nondescript, old but serviceable, if renovated. Special power lines would be needed, special sewage and water installations, environmental impact statements, city, county and state permits and the like.

These were not too formidable to obtain since other physician's offices were in the same area and a knowledgeable contractor would know how to handle these requirements. Of his options then, the most appealing was private pathology practice in a laboratory setting. He would need a loan from his banker. A tentative decision made, Hank changed into gym shoes and ran along the river path until he was tired. It was dark when he returned home.

He anticipated anything that moved in the dark shadows. Anyone who would attack in a large parking lot would be more successful with a surprise leap out of the shadows of the garage or bushes.

Entering his home was uneventful. Expecting not to sleep well, he took a hot shower and picked up the most boring reading articles he could find. These always served as the best soporific vehicle and without fail, he was asleep in five minutes.

Twenty

It was good that he slept well because the next morning, his chest was sore and both arms were painful. Also, he found he was in for a surprise.

Having always banked with one particular institution since his initial start in town, he was confident any building plans would be easily supported financially.

Rick Wilson, the bank manager greeted him warmly enough initially, but as soon as he began discussing his proposal and a loan, the banker's eyes began focusing on the wall behind him. Rick began to look uncomfortable, his replies became hesitant and his manner even became wary.

Something was wrong. Rick had never acted like this.

Then he remembered. Reliable Bank was the banker for the hospital and often a member of the bank was on the board of directors. Competition was competition. The board would not be receptive to any type of laboratory enterprise that would lessen hospital income.

Hank stopped describing his plans. "You're concerned because you're linked to the hospital."

"Well,...yes." Rick's words were slow and drawn out.

"Which means no to my proposal."

"I'm afraid so."

"Even though I've been with you for years?"

Rick shifted uncomfortably. "Could we make it a personal loan that was converted later...perhaps at some other bank? Your credit is good."

"True, but we're playing games, Rick. How do you handle other business borrowings—check first to see if it will interfere with the competition?"

Rick shifted even more uncomfortably in his chair. "No. I guess we don't...but in your case, Doctor, there are other factors that have been presented—some hospital committee has brought up your name..."

"...and put me on probation for my work?" He could feel the animosity rising. Any information that had gotten around would more than likely be misinterpreted.

"Well,...yes, something like that."

"Rick, I once read a banker quoted as saying that character made all the difference in loaning money. His name was J.P. Morgan. Has my character changed since you've known me?"

"No. I don't have anything against you personally."

"Then what's the problem?"

"Doc, I just can't." Rick had now hunkered down physically in his chair. It was almost a plea. Well, it was a plea. A problem pathologist he didn't need. It was no use hammering away at Rick. He took orders from others and he had his orders.

Hank left, disgusted and angry. St. Mary's Hospital was the fifth largest employer in the town. Their cash flow at the bank was huge. Every bank wanted the cash flow in their coffers. His own paltry accounts were expendable— just like he was expendable when he didn't hew to the line.

Troy Bank was a small competitor a few miles away. It was not affiliated with the hospital and was worth a try. Telephone first, he thought. It was easier and preferred by many bankers who liked to mull things over and check things out.

The telephone conversation went surprisingly well. He had an appointment that afternoon to discuss the general amount needed, the interest percentage, and type of repayment.

When Hank arrived, he was immediately ushered into the loan officer's room and greeted pleasantly. The entire transaction went smoothly and after minimal dickering, they settled on a reasonable percentage of interest, fifteen years, two points, drawn as needed during remodeling and then finalized for the full amount. It was quite a contrast to his reception at Reliable Bank.

As expected, Troy Bank wanted all his accounts immediately, including his trust accounts and CDs. It was only fair and Hank was almost pleased to change banks. He signed the necessary preliminary agreements and authorized transfers.

Hank contacted George Maisner, his contractor friend and racquet-ball partner, and discussed buying or leasing the property across the hospital at a reasonable sum. A preliminary inquiry only.

The nice thing about dealing with George Maisner was

that his whole family was involved in all stages of real estate. They could appraise, buy, sell, renovate, build-to-suit or whatever—all of it kept in the family.

Their prices were higher than usual but the workmanship was solid and the speedy way they operated was impressive. Even more impressive was the minimal amount of bickering that went on in the family. It was impossible for some jobs not to cross over into each other's territories, but the matters were settled quietly by George, who had enviably inherited a quiet but predictable good nature. For the first time, he felt happy and comfortable.

His beeper went off. He phoned in. It was the secretary to the president of St. Mary's, wanting to know if the rumors were true that he was resigning from the medical staff. Someone had planted the rumor. He didn't bother to answer. Another call was from the laboratory secretary, wanting to know what to do with his personal books and material.

So Rick Wilson, the banker, had alerted the hospital—he probably felt it was his duty as a director. Schmidt was losing no time in assisting the rumor. Whatever your enemy wanted, then the opposite should be implemented. That meant he should stay on. Corky had told him the easy way would be to quit.

He'd cancel his plans for moving—at least temporarily. Whatever Schmidt wanted would not be in his best interests.

Twenty-one

The police department sergeant called and asked him to drop back—the chief wanted to talk to him again. Hank walked to the police station, nodded to the desk sergeant, who now knew who he was, and started to walk on to the back room. The trustee was there with his offer of coffee again.

As he sipped the hot liquid, he noted the room was a sparse place with only a few mementos of the past. Bill Enzer had been around a long time. There had to be a good reason for the absence of mementos in his office. Some day, he'd ask. The chief came in and closed the door.

"What's he in for?" Hank asked, showing his coffee

mug. "Seems accommodating."

"Public nuisance. Chronic drunkenness. Makes good coffee."

The chief sat behind his desk and waited.

Hank found a hard-backed chair and sat down. Both understood that Monty would be part of the meeting. In a few quiet minutes, Monty arrived.

"Hi, Doc," offered Monty as a greeting. "What's new in the Haims case?"

"I thought you would tell me—you're investigating."

"We figured you'd be checking out your professional sources and tying down some loose ends that might be bothering you."

"Why would you think that?"

"Oh, our sources told us someone was making inquiries. Thought that might be you."

"I'm making a few inquiries, true. Nothing extensive. Just tying down loose ends—just as you say."

Monty grunted and waited. Hank waited. Waiting seemed to occupy a great deal of their meetings. Wasn't there a better ploy for obtaining information than just waiting and waiting and waiting?

Monty finally said, "Do you mind if we ask you some more questions about your relationship with Dr. Haims?"

"Okay, I guess. Do I have a choice?"

Monty didn't answer. He went to the chief's desk and shuffled some papers. When he found what he wanted, he grunted and read to himself slowly. Monty began asking questions as though they were written on the paper he was reading. Hank knew better. Monty had an enviable memory. The casualness of the interrogation went on but changed in tone as it expanded wider.

Suddenly, Monty looked up and said, "I understand you just got fired from the hospital here. Same reason you were put on probation?"

"You certainly obtain information fast. But it's incorrect. No. I haven't been fired. We had a difference of opinion on performing chemical tests with certain reagents. The probation had to do with something else—tissue reports that were supposedly inadequate."

"You got caught doin' lousy work, eh?"

Even knowing the purpose of the comment, it still hurt. Typical Monty. First, sweet talk. Friendliness. Flattery, even. Then the sudden jab and watchfulness for the reaction or overreaction. And they were...watching.

"Your way of getting a rise out of me stinks! You know the quality of my work," Hank heard himself say. His anger subsided with the outburst.

Monty grunted again. The chief shifted his position and stared through him without expression. The questions went on. And on.

"How much longer, guys?" Hank asked. The questions were getting tedious and repetitious. It was the usual attempt of trying to get a suspect to answer the same question in different ways and cross himself up. One small deviation is all they needed. Just one. In his case, how could it work?

Monty shrugged, looked at the chief, and then said, "Criticizing an autopsy protocol is easy for you—hindsight is infallible. How do we know what you've told us is true?"

"Why...check with a forensic pathologist," replied Hank. "Or has the body been cremated?"

"No," said the chief. "I've had the coroner put a halt on it. Who would you suggest redo the autopsy?"

"Joe Vinella or Don Markeley. One's in Wenachee and the other is in Seattle. Markeley can get away easier, since he's in private practice. You know it'll run twice the cost of the initial autopsy?"

The chief's smile disappeared. He was always at odds with the coroner who, as an elected official, used the cost factor as a platform for his election campaign. Whenever the coroner requested an autopsy, he insisted that all chemical analyses have his prior approval—which he gave very reluctantly.

"Would you call him now?" asked the chief.

Hank punched a few numbers on the telephone. Don's secretary tried to avoid giving him Don's private number—it was at the winery which had become an obsession with him at his nearby ranch in northern Idaho.

A voice that seemed to be experiencing some harassment answered in a half-shout. "*Yes!*"

"Tell me again," began Hank, "why someone who rarely drinks starts a winery from scratch...I can't comprehend the reasoning process."

"Sheer idiocy is the answer! Total, unequivocal stupidity! Whipple! Is that you?"

"Yep. Chief Enzer needs a forensic job done. Know anyone qualified?" Markeley was taught by Dr. Helpern in the New York City Medical Examiner's Office—an irreverent-genius type, he was more than qualified.

"I'm available."

"Now?"

Don was accepting too readily. His venture into the commercial winery had to be eating up his salary.

"Now."

"Which means those old vats you bought at a bargain from the winery in France are springing leaks." Silence. Hank waited for the blood to stop flowing.

"Anyone tell you you're nothing but a cold, analytical bastard, Whipple? A know-it-all smartass?"

"No. I mean, it's the first time today. See you early A.M.?"

"Make it seven. It'll take me two hours to drive down."

Hank looked at the chief, who nodded. "Seven it is."

Don held on. "How come *you're* not doing the post?"

"A member of our department did it."

"Must be the young guy they hired. He kick you out of the department yet and take over?"

Hank winced. "Funny how I can see the humor in your wine vats leaking but none in discussing department politics."

"I'm sure!" said Don Markeley. "That's why I'm in private practice!"

Hank handed the phone over to the chief for the discussion of details.

"I guess that means you can go," said the chief, pleasantly but clearly indicating he wanted a private conversation with Dr. Markeley. Certainly part of it would be asking Don to confirm what Hank had told him.

Hank took the empty coffee cup out to the trustee. The one bright spot at the police station. "Good coffee. Thanks!"

The trustee grinned his appreciation. "I'm here so often I'm like a permanent employee," he said. "Come again when you can stay longer. A lot longer."

He then laughed and laughed at his joke.

Twenty-two

Don Markeley was at the lab the next morning, on time as promised, with his black bag. The chief and Monty were waiting.

Markeley said, "I've notified Dr. Schmidt that I've been requested to perform a second post-mortem exam on the body of Dr. John Haims. He declined to be present, so I guess we will proceed."

Don had performed his ethical duty and was the pure professional now. No small talk or bantering. No witticisms.

After Don had examined the brain at the morgue, they went to the funeral home and were ushered in by a sleepy, put-upon embalmer who immediately asked how soon the body could be cremated.

"We'll let you know," was Markeley's curt answer. Markeley held no appreciation for body preparation work by morticians.

Once he set up his dictating machine with its foot pedal, he began his comments with the time, day, mortician's name who identified the body and the persons present observing the autopsy. Normal procedure.

He then reviewed the pictures at the scene and quickly read through the police report and Schmidt's report. He sliced through Schmidt's stitches, opened the plastic bag and laid out each organ, comparing the report with what he was observing. He began taking pictures, concentrating on the fracture lines of the skull and subcutaneous skin hemorrhages.

It was oddly comforting to Hank to watch Don work. Without deviation, Don followed his own protocol, like a checklist before flying an airplane. Nothing would be left to chance. Every mark would be photographed and a comment would be made as to its pre-mortem or post-mortem cause. He never forgot the essentials.

In about two hours, he was through. His filled jars and vials went into his black bag—all in appropriate places. Blood, bile, stomach contents, large segments of liver and spleen were all bottled or placed in heavy plastic to be frozen. He had obtained samples of skin around the entrance wounds and in the path through the skull bone. Since the excised bladder contained no urine, he washed the bladder with distilled water and saved this fluid, too.

Hank felt warm satisfaction in watching a colleague work and waited for a twinge of envy to appear. It didn't. Hank felt surprise that it wasn't like being envious of Keith and his athletic or running ability.

Both police officers had watched the whole procedure silently.

The chief said, "Thanks for coming down, Don."

Don? he had said. What was this? Hank looked at them both. "You know each other?" Hank asked.

"Why sure," grinned the chief.

It all fell into place. Don Markeley had been his choice to recheck the autopsy, only the chief had finessed it so that Hank had agreed that a second look was necessary and suggested the names of forensic pathologists. That way, Chief Enzer had more ammunition when the coroner objected to the extra charges.

Don Markeley looked at his watch and grunted. "See you." He drove away, breaking the speed limit in town within the first fifteen seconds of departure.

The chief winced as he followed the disappearing vehicle with his eyes and said, half to himself, "I don't know how he manages that without getting a bunch of tickets."

"He collects them and uses them for wallpaper," Hank replied. "I know. Ever see his office in Seattle? A whole wall!"

Twenty-three

Arriving home, he checked the mail. There were the usual large number of drug advertisements, seminars and workshop offerings.

He thought about the Haims autopsy. There were unusual discrepancies in its performance by Schmidt. Why? The usual protocol wasn't being followed, it had been hurried early in the morning and things were left out—perhaps like President Kennedy's autopsy—on purpose or due to ineptness?

The skull fracture in the occiput—the back part of the head. Direction of the trajectory. Angles? Not useful here. Analysis of the blood splatter from the wound. Direction of the drops. Toxicology. Absent. Why? This was a routine procedure.

He decided to take a walk. It turned bleak and cold that evening. The wind blew a continuous wave of debris through the streets in several different directions without pause.

He intended to enjoy the air regardless of the ever-present wind but the chill factor was not enjoyable, so he gave up and returned home. Corky was still gone and the empty house seemed so strange without all the usual sounds. He tried to convince himself it was restful but it wasn't true; the noisy activity was necessary.

He had plenty of time to reflect on the murder of Dr. Haims. If Haims was arrogant and heavy-handed here, then he must have been the same elsewhere—at school, during internship and residency and during practice. Some-one who cheats here must have cheated before...and per-haps got caught.

Something that had harmed someone—enough to cause that person such anger that he would kill. But murder? It was deeper than just a grudge.

Hank thought about homicide gunshot wounds in general. Over sixty percent occurred between relatives or close acquaintances and were solved fairly quickly. The difficult cases to solve were the one time crimes, never to be repeated, like the gunshots into cars on the highways by psychopaths. Unless witnesses were present or the psycho's buddies tattled, tracing the act to the person was extremely difficult.

Women almost never used guns or knives on their victims. Poisoning, yes. Occasionally sharp objects such as needles and knives but rarely hatchets and axes. That probably left out Mrs. Haims, who alleged she hated guns. But how would one know this was the truth? He could assume Monty had checked out the truthfulness of that statement. He called Corky several times, being careful not to mention anything about the lab and his future plans. It was easier to talk about the horses and the action at the Roundup Grounds. The children were enjoying the change.

That behind him, he was free to concentrate on finding Haims's murderer, using every afternoon and evening.

Twenty-four

It was 7:30 A.M. the next morning and time for the first surgery. It would be a short day since Alex had agreed to cover his afternoons so he could get on with his investigation.

Hank put his feet up on the desk and reviewed the schedule sheet typed up by the secretaries the previous evening. His legs muscles never stopped getting sore. Racquet-ball muscles were different than the horseback riding muscles. One set became accustomed and the other unaccustomed. Tomorrow it would be the back muscles again.

Scheduled were three consults with frozen sections.

Frozen sections of the surgical tissue enabled the pathologist to render an opinion immediately instead of making
the surgeon wait until the next day. The three scheduled
consultations were for Sam Sager—one after the other:
breast, neck nodes and bowel. In addition, there was a fine
needle aspiration of the thyroid and a bone marrow interpretation as well as the usual appointments with lab supervisors.

No. He had forgotten. The supervisors were now
reporting to Dr. Schmidt. Hank felt a twinge of loss even
though the supervisors related mostly complaints and
problems that had to be resolved. Well, he sighed, that left
the other work. He had to get cracking on his main
concern.

Sam Sager had acquired Haims's surgical patients.
Although he was not Haims's partner, he was in the same
building and the two surgeons were forced to spell one
another on weekends. Dr. Haims had the greater number
of patients. Why he did was a puzzle since Sam had equal
skills, a far more pleasant manner, and being a humorist
and a great storyteller didn't hurt.

The call came from surgery and he went down to the
frozen section room. The breast biopsy was in a green
plastic bowl. Surrounded by light-yellow fat, a small, hard,
encapsulated nodule was within the excised tissue.

Hank felt it, cut it and diagnosed "Fibroadenoma.
Benign."

Not too long ago, it would have been sufficient to
simply give the diagnosis to the surgeon but now, in the
awakened litigious society, Schmidt insisted on viewing
everything through the microscope. The other two pathologists had changed their routines and did the same. He
would conform by cutting the tumor thinly, staining it and
placing the thin tissue on a glass slide. Then he would

confirm it by looking at it through the microscope.

He called the surgeon in the operating room. "Whipple here. Looks like a benign fibroadenoma, Dr.Sager. I'll freeze it and get back to you in a few minutes."

"Thank you, Hank."

Just then Schmidt rushed in, breathless, his mustache quivering. "Did you do the frozen yet? I have to check you, you know. Tissue surgery rules."

Hank stepped back. "Didn't you see the consult reports from Seattle? They agreed with my diagnoses."

Schmidt hesitated. "There are no orders from the committee," he said lamely. "Until they cancel their directives—"

Dr. Sager walked into the room, still clad in the green operating gown, his surgical hat typically askew.

"It's consistent with a benign fibroadenoma, Dr. Sager," said Schmidt eagerly.

The surgeon glared at Schmidt. "Hell, I know that. Hank told me that five minutes ago over the intercom. I've already closed."

"Well...a frozen still has to be done."

Sager looked at Hank. "Thanks for letting me get on with it," he said. "When you have several surgeries to go, you appreciate a quick report."

Sam Sager turned to Schmidt. "He saves me time by reading it grossly. While I'm closing the skin, he confirms it with the frozen. Now I can dictate the operative report and they can clean the room for the next patient. Why don't you do what he does?"

Sam Sager lumbered out.

"There are two more surgical consults for Dr. Sager," Hank said. "Are you going to come back for those too or are you going to wait for them here?"

Schmidt's mustache twitched. "I'm only abiding by the

committee directive. It wasn't my idea."

"How about the fine-needle aspirations?"

"Who are the doctors?"

"What difference does that make?"

Schmidt turned and walked out in his distinctive waddle without answering.

The rest of the morning went quickly. Again, Hank made sure he spent some time between surgeries waiting in the surgical lounge where the physicians gathered. Any knowledge he could pick up might have a bearing on the murder. Nursing the third cup of coffee of the morning, Hank felt the atmosphere was now reasonably friendly—a distinct difference from the previous days when he had been tolerated and even ignored.

"Hi, Hank," said Dr. French, the neurologist. Another doctor smiled and nodded at him. Things were normal.

A few of the quality assurance committee members came and left the surgical lounge. They were neither friendly nor unfriendly. Only a few deliberately ignored him and, as expected, Dr. Span was one. He expected that as time went on, Span would ease into a superficial friendliness and any of the ugly statements that he had made under the guidance of Dr. Haims would be forgotten. The minutes of the quality assurance committee meeting would disappear.

Dr. Sam Sager was still waiting for his next patient to be readied in the surgical room. He had taken off his surgical cap and the gray streaks accented the sides of his straight black hair.

"Don't see you hanging around the parking lot these days," he laughed.

Hank shook his head and thanked him for the rescue and his kind words in the frozen section room in surgery.

Sam waved off the thanks and sat down heavily in the

chair opposite.

Unlike Haims, Sam Sager liked eating well and often—looks be damned, his abdomen hung over his belt. His plaid L. L. Bean shirt was open and his shoes had ruffled soles—all for comfort. He was in a typical jovial mood and apparently had nothing on his mind; the conversation seemed to drift aimlessly.

"Hope they catch that bugger. Did you irritate somebody recently? Other than the usual surgeons?" Sam smiled.

"Well... yes, come to think of it. I had just finished telling the salesman for Hempter Reagents that they weren't any good."

Sam looked thoughtful. "That rings a bell. Hempter? Something about...during training, I remember something... What was it now?"

"Don't tell me they go around beating up anyone who refuses to use their products."

"Yeah! I remember now! The competition. I bandaged up a salesman for another company that got beat up. The bones healed but he refused the territory after that. No proof, of course, but he insisted it was Hempter."

Hank shrugged. "I got off easy, then."

Sam smiled. "By the way, I understand you didn't do the autopsy on Haims."

"That's right. Dr. Schmidt did the post-mortem."

"Was it suicide?" Sam tilted his head slightly and looked at him through a squint of his eyes.

"Police are investigating other probabilities—homicide is uppermost in their minds."

Sam groaned. "Haims was a moody person with deep antagonisms, many of which didn't make sense. I know. I spelled him for vacations. They did rule out suicide, you say?"

"I believe they did. But the investigation continues."

"Haims liked to read, you know." Sam continued to muse. "Easy to pick off a person who has regular habits like reading every evening at the same time. Could happen to any of us."

Hank nodded and then something hit the back of his mind when Dr. Sager made that statement. Perhaps it was the comment about reading—Sam knew Haims's habits. What else did he know? Hank tried not to change expression with his question. "Was he well-liked by his colleagues?" asked Hank, trying to make it sound like an innocent question. "Stuck in the lab as we are, we rarely see interactions between physicians."

"Well," blustered Dr. Sam, shifting his eyes and weight at the same time. "Haims had his good points and bad points; good days and bad days. He was a man of extremes—constant hates but mild likes. We had our arguments."

"Did he ever operate on you or your family?" Hank didn't know why he phrased the question. It just popped out. Where did that question come from?

Sam was startled. "Oh, no! That would be too close to home. No. It's not a good idea to have someone you know well operate on your own family, because you would be second-guessing the surgeon all the way."

Why did Hank ask the question? There had to be a subconscious reason why it surfaced. Why? Because...he wanted to see if Sam would deliberately lie about his feelings toward Haims.

Haims had operated on one of Sam's children and it was a bad result. Not only was the simple fracture poorly set, but the cast was put on too tight. Circulation to the limb was cut off with resulting nerve damage and, to make matters worse, the skin ulcerated and an anaerobic infection developed.

In short, a simple procedure became a nightmare. Osteomyelitis and septicemia set in and the blood poisoning advanced so rapidly that it was terrifying to watch. Hank had worked with the bacteriology department and cultured out the organism. They found the exact antibiotics that would kill the germs. At least the child's life was saved.

But her arm was gone.

Sam Sager would not forget that particular episode of illness. He had lied for a reason. Was this casual visit also for a reason? Was his expressed appreciation during the frozen section also done for a reason? Was Sam maneuvering?

Sam adroitly changed the subject and was talking about the three patients he had operated on that morning and their individual problems. Sam was able to make everything amusing with his witty observations and humor.

"Lady's husband came home from work and she greeted him with, 'I've got good new and bad news. Which do you want to hear first?' 'The good news!' he said. 'The air bag works,' she offered."

In spite of his suspicions, Hank enjoyed hearing the anecdotes and laughed. Then Sam made his special swinging wave and left.

Twenty-five

The two other biopsies went quickly. The lymph nodes were not cancerous and the bowel tumor already was felt to be highly suspicious for malignancy. Hank confirmed that it was indeed an adenocarcinoma—a type of cancer involving the inner lining of the large colon.

The fine-needle aspirations started with a thyroid nodule. Stackle, a surgeon, decided to perform it himself but wanted Hank to assist.

The patient was a twenty-five-year-old girl who was very animated. She talked through the entire procedure, apologizing every few minutes for her continuous conversation. Stackle was a pleasant surgeon who did most of his work at the other hospital across the river. It was a relaxing surgery because Stackle only grinned and said over and over how much he preferred her conversation to worry and fear over the procedure.

Hank took the smears and stained them with Quick-Stain to confirm that the amount and type of tissue was sufficient for microscopic evaluation diagnosis. Happily, the thyroid aspirations were benign colloid cysts. Everyone was pleased at the benign result.

The next patient was a pleasant, anxious college student with a normal white blood count, but anemia and a low number of platelets. The attending physician was suspicious and had ordered a bone marrow examination. A medication reaction? Too often, medications caused untoward reactions in the body, especially the blood forming centers. But the patient was on no medicines whatever.

The student's main complaint was that recently he had become short of breath jogging three miles when he had previously completed five miles without any difficulty. The accompanying slip read: "Eight grams of hemoglobin. Forty thousand platelets." That was enough. The normal white blood count could be discounted as could the normal differential. Leukemia occurred with a low white count, a normal white count or, what was more usual, a high white count.

Hank talked to the student and explained what he was going to do. Using the usual sterile procedure, he prepared the skin with iodine, cleaned it with alcohol and injected 2 percent Xylocaine through the skin and down to the periosteum which covered the bone. After a short wait, Hank aspirated some marrow from the iliac crest into the syringe.

The marrow did not come easily. A bad sign. Usually a quick suction into a 20-cc syringe would obtain abundant marrow material. He made another attempt in a different area through the same skin incision. This time a small amount of marrow was obtained. It might not be sufficient for a diagnosis.

Rather than discharge the patient and have him return again, Hank injected five mg of Valium intravenously and waited fifteen minutes. After checking that the student's pain reaction was blunted, he obtained a core of marrow.

"I'm sorry for this extra procedure," Hank said, "but it will save time doing it now rather than having you come back again. Did it hurt very much?"

"Well...I could feel it. Like the kick of a mule. But..."

Patients differed in their pain perceptions. The intravenous Valium was better than the Xylocaine alone and sometimes he added an eighth of a grain of morphine to the anesthesia to achieve satisfactory dulling of the pain.

If the marrow was replaced with leukemic cells or filled with primitive parasitic white cells, a bone marrow aspiration was difficult. He handed the material to the technologist who made smears, kept a clot for sectioning and placed part of the bone biopsy into formalin for decalcification and later sectioning. Special enzyme stains and chromosome studies of the malignant cells not only classified the leukemia but also aided in the prognosis.

Later that morning at the lab, he read the initial stained slides and phoned the physician the preliminary finding: Acute myelogenous leukemia. He set the slide to one side for their 3:30 P.M. conference.

The rest of the morning went quickly. When he returned to the office, the lab secretary said Mrs. Haims wanted to talk to him.

Hank picked up the phone. "Dr. Whipple?" An angry voice.

"Yes, speaking."

"My name is Martha Haims. You are investigating the death of my husband and are harassing me and my family. I want it to stop!"

"The police are investigating the death, Mrs. Haims. The pathologist only—"

"I know what a pathologist does! They're wrong and you're wrong in this case to keep questioning the doctor's death. Our family is not involved!"

She spoke of him as "the doctor." Not as "my husband" or as "John." It spoke volumes of their relationship.

"Yes, Mrs. Haims. I don't know about your family being implicated by the—"

"Yes, my son is! One of you discussed the case with other doctors and it was reported to me. My son has gone through some difficult times, but that has all been behind us. Now this type of innuendo has got to stop!"

"I'm sorry, Mrs. Haims. You'll have to believe me, but I know nothing about your son and could not have said anything."

"Then who did?"

"I've no idea."

"Someone did. Who is in charge in your department? The remarks came out of the laboratory pathologist."

"Dr. Schmidt is in charge. He also did the post-mortem on your husband."

"Could you transfer me, please? I'd like to talk to him."

"Gladly, Mrs. Haims. I'm going to put you on hold. You won't hear anything during the transfer of the call, so don't hang up."

"Thank you."

Hank hummed to himself while he transferred the phone call to Dr. Schmidt. As department head, Hank had always received the brunt of criticism. How pleasant it was to share true responsibility with others.

Twenty-six

Mrs. Haims's call threw up more interesting facets to the murder. A mother always saw a son blemish-free. To admit to a stranger that her son had gone through "difficult times" was indeed of interest to everyone concerned about the death. Did "difficult times" mean drugs, alcohol, teenage rebelliousness or something more serious? Haims kept things hushed up so Hank only heard hints of problems.

Who would know? The police chief. Also, Don Markeley's autopsy report should be finished by now. The chief had that, too.

Hank dropped the preliminary bone marrow smear interpretations on the desk of the typist and signed out to

Alex.

He went to the police station, hoping the chief would be there. He was told the chief was busy.

"Coffee?" The trustee was new but eager. This one had a battered face with several lacerations which looked as though he had been in a fight.

"Thanks. How'd you get so banged up? Police brutality?"

The trustee stopped smiling at the horror of the idea. "No. No! They're the greatest here. I'm trying for a permanent job."

"Sure." It was his turn to smile.

"Come in, doc," Chief Enzer was typically curt.

"You may not like why I'm here. Do you have Dr. Markeley's report? I'd like some information."

"Answer: No. Information: Need an encyclopedia?"

"Less than that will do. Haims's son. How old is he? What's he gotten into besides the usual kid stuff with keggers and traffic tickets?"

"What made you ask about him?"

"Only curiosity. Chief…do you always answer a question with a question? What are you like off-duty?"

"Compared to whom?"

This was an old joke. The chief once had a police officer in his department who always answered every question with, "Compared to whom?" or, "Compared to what?" This got tedious quite quickly when you asked, "How are you?" and received as an answer, "Compared to whom?" Even the officer's family was not exempt. When someone asked him, "How's your family?" the answer came back, "Compared to?"

"How is 'Compared to whom?' these days. Haven't seen him around," asked Hank.

"Moved on. We couldn't take his comparisons any

longer."

"That is very understandable. Tell me about Haims's son. The problem one."

"Why?"

"Suspects are always checked out in a definite order: spouse, heirs, family, friends, acquaintances and, in this case, patients. You've checked on him early," Hank said. A positive statement.

"Yes. Well…the best thing to be said about him is that he was a methodical type. He tried out everything without missing anything listed or unlisted. First the alcohol, then medicines from his dad's office—some he sold and some he used himself, uppers and downers, heavy stuff and mixtures of all of them.

"Detox?"

"Several times."

"And…violence?"

"What do you think?"

"Haims spent a good deal of time pushing high morals on the rest of us. I'd like to think something positive came out of his insistence on setting an example."

"You'd be wrong. Kid had too many assault records. When last seen, he was traveling down the road, alone, heading for California."

"They all seem to go to California."

"Better there than here." The chief leaned back in his chair at the thought. "Mother was a tiger about him. The drugs, assault and battery cases, thefts—always was someone else's fault."

"Think he came back?"

"That's what we've been working on. Haims and his son were continually battling with each other. If you're asking whether the son is a suspect, the answer is yes. Tracer is out on him."

"Thanks. That is what I wanted to know." Hank left. The dark, dreary hall he walked down had only one dull yellow light. Taxpayers' money was also being saved on wall paint.

The trustee was behind him, calling for Hank's attention. "I got beat up in a fight. Nothing to do with the police. Honest! It was a fight!" The trustee thought a moment and grinned. "I lost."

"Too bad."

"Oh, no! I was lucky! If I'd a won, they'd a tossed me in jail!"

The toothless trustee laughed and laughed at his own joke. The sound reverberated down the dismal hall as Hank walked out the door. Were all these drunks humorists?

Twenty-seven

In the surgery lounge, Keith, the anesthesiologist, sought him out and asked about autopsies. "I'm going to court about a child that died, a Mongolian child who aspirated after a tonsillectomy. A question came up during the interrogatory regarding edema of the brain. How can you detect excess fluid?"

The question was sensible enough. Usually the tonsillar pillars, edges of the cerebellum, show a compression line as did the uncus area located at the bottom sides of the brain. The brain surfaces, gyri, are swollen and the infoldings, sulci, are compressed. Those factors alone indicate increased cerebrospinal fluid pressure was present even if excess fluid and dilated ventricles are not obvious at post-mortem.

"It must be hard tracing out what happened in certain cases—especially those involving suicide and murder." Keith had changed the subject.

"Yes," Hank said. "It is not only difficult but sometimes impossible. A certain percentage have to be listed under the category of unresolved, because there is no anatomic factor. Highly suspect, of course, is cardiac arrhythmia."

"How is Haims's case coming along?"

"Dr. Schmidt performed the autopsy."

"I hear another pathologist came down and redid it."

"Yes. The police chief wanted another opinion."

"Something wrong?"

"I guess he thought so."

Keith looked directly at Hank for a moment. He seemed a bit agitated—surgery must not have gone well that morning. Turning his back for a moment, Keith grabbed a piece of fruit from the food plate and bit into it.

He remarked, "Haims was not that well-liked, you know. Any idea who do did it?"

"I don't know."

This answer seemed to upset the anesthesiologist. He felt Hank was holding back. Nothing irritated a fellow doctor more than to have opinions or facts withheld. It was like being told you couldn't be trusted.

Keith expressed his irritation. "You guys always have definite ideas. Why don't you ever let the rest of us in on it? You helped bring in the other pathologist, Markeley, and you even checked on everyone's school records and places we practiced!"

"Sorry, Keith," said Hank. "It's not deliberate. Can't comment on something that could go to court. Any smart lawyer would make a lot of points with the jury by trying to get a doctor to admit that he gossiped about a case with everyone."

"True. True." Keith had a chagrined look on his face. He had blurted out too much.

"What made you think I checked out Haims and others?"

"You did, didn't you?"

"Maybe. Tell me."

Keith smiled for the first time as though he had penetrated a secret. "Easy. I figured it this way. You're an uptight, circumspect character. Knowing that and knowing Haims cut you down, indirectly, in quality assurance committee—don't look surprised at me—everybody knows Span jumps to whatever tune Haims plays—so that you're no longer department head...Well, it's no feat of imagination that after he dies, you'll come under suspicion...So, you check up on Haims and everyone to clear yourself. Besides, a friend of mine called to say a pathologist was asking detailed questions about me and the family."

"What are you doing in anesthesiology when you're making so many Sherlockian deductions about your fellow doctors?"

"Enjoyed pathology. It was my next choice in school. I still wonder if I did the right thing—and I keep up on a lot of the literature. But the idea of doing autopsies..." Keith shuddered.

Just then, the loudspeaker paged Keith for Room D. A nurse anesthetist had a problem with a patient in the operating room. Keith gave Hank a wink and with a triumphant smile, he kept a pointed finger on Hank as he moved away, knowing he had scored. Hank wondered how many others knew what Keith knew as he returned to his office.

Suspects were Haims's family, with the son an open

question. Then came the strange hurry-up, early-morning autopsy by Dr. Schmidt which left out important findings. Then Dr. Sam Sager, who benefitted from acquiring Dr. Haims's patients, coming in to discuss Haims. Sam was untruthful about Haims operating on his family. Why?

Keith Gray seemed to know more than usual about Haims. Was this merely idle curiosity? He seemed unusually knowledgeable about the extent of activities surrounding the Haims case and his wife, Darlene, was excessively agitated about Haims's death.

Haims's patients? Was there someone who was so stressed out about the results of surgery that he killed the surgeon? The ancient Code of Hammurabi was necessary in those times and a doctor who injured an eye or limb of a patient had his own eye of limb equally injured or cut out.

But Haims was generally so slick with his patients. Hank didn't know anyone who felt injured except Cliff Evers. If they did, they kept it quiet.

How violent could someone like Cliff Evers be? Cliff knew Haims was lying to him about his hormone levels. Would he blame Haims for the breakup of his marriage?

Dr. Schmidt was the only one who appeared friendly to Dr. Haims but Haims had been unselective in his nastiness. It was a matter of time before Haims would turn his wrath on someone. Was there a long-smoldering hatred by Schmidt for being ridiculed in front of others?

Something vital was left out. A piece of information was absent or being overlooked that could lead to the killer. Was there a connection between altered records and Haims's death? What were the actual facts as of now? He began to go over the same suspects and motives.

His friends were not concerned about hospital politics and no physician really cared who ran the pathology department. Each had problems of their own.

Don's report may help, he told himself wearily. What the chief is uncovering may open it all up—but it's taking so long!

He drove downtown. The Bolli was filled with the usual group. Conversation was animated. The voices overlayed each other.

"Stop smoking! How many times do I have to stomp it out for you until you learn."

"Hey…don't tell him just to quit. Tell him to switch to something else I can make money on." Bill and his brother sold tobacco and sweets. It was a fifty-year-old business— their father having been one of the town fathers.

"If you can work up a story that the judge has never heard before, it'll get you off every time. Let me tell you what happened last week in police court…" Police court was right across the street and the public was allowed to sit in on the proceedings. Even under oath, people allowed their imaginations to run rampant in explaining why they had been arrested. It was like listening to your teenage child explaining why he was arriving home at 3:30 A.M.

"The mill is going to cut back. They're not buying any material right now and have let the part-timers go." This was bad news.

Zack, the acknowledged clown of the group, spied him and his face lit up with pleasure. "Come on over, Whipple. Tell us how you did away with Haims and confused the chief. Is it true you did the autopsy yourself? Give us all the gory details. Don't leave out anything! The boys want to hear it *all*. Too bad I have to leave right now. They'll fill me in later…but I hope not."

Typical Zack. He always took some true facts and twisted them so that they ended in a humorous but embarrassing conclusion.

"Thanks, Zack." Hank appreciated the jibe. "You know

the chief won't let a word out about his suspicions until…bang, you're looking from the inside out."

He looked over at the chief, who smiled slightly and nodded. Hank added, "When were you going to pick up Zack for all those parking tickets, Chief? Pay up fast, Zack. It's better from the outside looking in. Take my word for it…On second thought, don't take my word for it. Why not try a weekend in the tank? I have it on very good authority that it's an experience you'll never forget."

The tank was a large enclosure in the basement of the police station which was in use because of the shortage of jail space. There were no facilities except a pot in the corner. All drunks, junkies, psychopaths and unknowns of all types who did not appear violent were placed there temporarily while being booked or until they were identified. The only problem was predicting who was violent and who wasn't. In such claustrophobic surroundings, even the mildest person could become goaded into a fury and too often, fights broke out, resulting in a trip to the hospital.

Zack pretended to consider the offer and knit his eyebrows. "Free meals included, Chief?"

"For you, we'll even add peanut butter sandwiches."

"Well," said Zack, going out the door, "it's the best offer I've had so far today, and if that's the way the day's going to keep going, I'm in deep, deep trouble."

Twenty-eight

The morning hospital work finished, he signed out to Alex again. Leafing through his notes, Hank made a phone call.

Keith Gray's wife answered the telephone. "I'm sorry, but he's not here. He'll be back in about an hour. He said he was going to run down to the river and back."

She took the message and it was approximately an hour when Keith returned the call.

"I'd like to see you," Hank said without any preliminaries.

"Sure. Something serious or can it wait?"

"It could wait, but it's better discussed tonight."

They agreed on a bar near Keith's home that was rarely crowded.

"Never met with a pathologist at night before. Must be a real problem if you need to talk right now." Keith was pleasant as always but curiously wary.

"Right."

They got their drinks. Hank had a whiskey and Keith ordered plain 7-Up. They held back their conversation until they sat down in a corner booth. It was a another gloomy night. Even the booth light cast gloomy shadows.

Hank started. "The police chief wants the information I've been able to canvass—about Dr. Haims and all his contacts."

"Why tell me about this?" Keith looked down at his drink and then back up.

"Your name cropped up in those background checks I made—as you know it would."

Keith looked casual. "So."

"So..., you and Haims worked together at the same hospital. Not only that, but you had a warm social relationship then."

Keith shifted his body and looked at his drink. "True."

"The relationship obviously abruptly ended."

Keith looked thoughtful. "Yes."

"Something happened that caused the sudden break."

"Could be." Keith was now wary and interested.

"That something was a disaster to you and your family."

"It was a long time ago. A long time ago."

Hank paused. "But not long enough to be forgotten."

"No."

"Do you want to tell me about it or shall I try to piece it all together from the information I've got?"

"Not much to tell. Surgery was necessary on our child.

Haims did it. The child died. One of those things that happen. Only it happened to us."

The words were spoken lightly but Keith looked suddenly haggard. Was it the adrenalin from his long run that was flowing away? Or was it something else?

"There was more to it than that, Keith. The surgery was a simple tonsillectomy. It was done on a Friday morning. The child began to bleed Saturday afternoon. Dr. Haims didn't work on Saturday, his Sabbath. He turned the case over to a new resident. The resident thought he had stopped the bleeding. He assured you that he had. You were kept so busy elsewhere that when you finally saw your child, she was bled out. Dr. Haims was called but either couldn't be reached or refused to come in. The information is hazy about that part—but he wasn't available. Blood was ordered stat. The bleeding finally stopped and the child was discharged.

"About three months later, a worse case scenario developed. The blood was contaminated with non-A, non-B virus—the virus we now call C—no test was available at that time in any blood bank. Acute hepatitis, then liver failure and finally the worst of nightmares: the delta virus became superimposed on the non-A, non-B virus infection and the liver became necrotic. A liver transplant was attempted. The baby died. All for a minor tonsillectomy."

"The bastard wouldn't come in. He was available," muttered Keith.

"Haims was in the clear, technically. His agreement with the hospital staff was that he would be unavailable Saturdays. He blamed the resident surgeon. The resident resigned and blamed the blood bank. The blood bank blamed the unavailability of any testing for non-A non-B virus. So, since the blood bank belonged to the hospital, your employer, they took the ultimate blame. Not that you would have cared about that or where the blame lay. The end result was that your wife, Darlene, became *non compos mentis* for months."

Keith reached up with both hands and rubbed his face and eyes. He didn't speak for a few minutes.

Hank felt like a sadist. He was forcing Keith to relive the agonizing slow death of his child, watching the child's skin turn a deeper and deeper yellow as its mind became more and more obtuse. Then coma. Convulsions. Death.

"Your next question is whether I killed Haims after all these years? Couldn't I have done it before? I would have had plenty of opportunity."

"I don't know. I'm just presenting a strong motive to you."

"And that's what you've basically discovered?"

"Yes."

"If you suspect me of shooting Haims, then you'll find out about Darlene. She is a crack shot with a pistol...competed for prizes and won a lot of them. Had a father who wanted a boy; Darlene ended up an only child, so he pushed her into male activities and competitions. Anybody else have a strong motive besides us?"

Hank tried to break the tension. "My reasons for all these questions—myself. Dr. Haims changed my pathology diagnoses to suit his own purposes."

"Meaning he wanted to avoid surveillance by the tissue surgery committee. All surgeons would like to do that. How could he change the diagnosis? The true copy would be in your permanent file. You'd have him there!"

"The hospital file that matters is in the patient's chart. He bribed or cajoled a record room typist to change just the diagnosis. As you know, today, the trend in pathology is to leave out the microscopic description of the tissue report and only give the diagnosis itself. That makes it easy to wipe out the correct diagnosis—appendix—and substitute acute appendicitis; normal gall bladder can easily be changed to acute cholecystitis. It is a simple matter of using liquid eraser, retyping and Xeroxing the original—destroying the incriminating original and filing the new original in the patient's chart."

"And that way, a computer search for normal tissue removal by surgeons would be nil."

"Right. At least with Haims's surgeries and a few of his close buddies."

"When did you find out about it? Knowing you, you probably confronted him," Keith reflected. "That's when he began poor-mouthing you and having committees formed investigating your work. I remember when he started in on you—he began discussing your incompetent diagnoses in the operating room."

Hank blinked. "Normal procedure for surgeons to bait pathologists or complain about them. Haims was very persuasive and being chairman of the tissue surgery committee cinched it. He suggested as much to me during the confrontation."

"So you became a suspect because he got you demoted and had you lined out to be fired." Keith smiled a rueful smile and nodded to himself. "You'll have to admit that there is something amusing about a pathologist being the suspect when he is used to incriminating others all the time."

"It is a different experience. Yes." Hank smiled.

Keith twisted his empty glass. "You're turning this information over to the police in the morning—is that it?"

"Yes. I thought I'd tell you about the incriminating material in it. We've been friends for a long time. You'd do the same for me."

"Yes. That I would." Keith lowered his eyes to his glass.

"Think I'll have a Scotch."

"I'll join you."

Fifteen minutes later, they parted.

Keith had actually admitted nothing more except that he could have had the opportunity to kill Haims on many previous occasions.

But then, so could have many others.

Hank felt partially relieved. But he now knew whose picture was in the locket Darlene wore around her neck.

Nothing was forgotten.

Twenty-nine

The next morning, Dr. Schmidt was absent. Pathologists are always on duty in the mornings for surgery consultations. The secretaries were told only that he would not be in—no reason.

There were important problems with seriously ill patients. Decisions had to be made. Opinions formulated and confirmed, then rendered to the attending physician.

The Pap smears took several hours to review, even though they had been screened by the cytologists. Anyone could have a bad day and miss a cell. And one cell is all it took to diagnose a dysplastic or cancerous condition. Screeners were helpful but not infallible.

Body fluids were the hardest, partly because there was no information accompanying the material. Hank learned never to read out the fluids without some background knowledge.

He set aside the body fluid slides as a group and went to the patient wards to check the charts. After making notes on each case, he returned to the microscope and began reading the Pap smears and the centrifuged "buttons" of material from the body fluids. Two were cancers. Two were atypical and the patient needed further clinical evaluation. Five were normal.

The fine-needle aspirations, or FNAs as they were called, attracted a special interest. It was an early pet project because it meant minimal trauma to the patient and maximal results. Hopefully. But a negative result on an FNA was of no value. It meant only that no malignant cells were present in that particular area where the cells were sucked out. Only a positive reading on an FNA was significant. And that really became a technical problem of obtaining a true sampling of the "lump" from the surgeon. Since surgeons' techniques differed, some pathologists performed their own FNAS on patients for that reason.

Hank made phone calls to the doctors involved who had sent in tissues and gave them a provisional report. Then to the oncologists to prepare them for the unusual cases they would soon be treating. The malignant diagnoses he again placed in the conference room for routine review.

"I saw Dr. Schmidt down at the police station this morning." Darrel Sims was always interested in any unusual occurrence that involved the lab personnel.

"Oh."

"I had to drop off a few bucks on a parking ticket. Our lab courier—not me," Darrel hastened to add.

Hank nodded. "Sure. Not you, Darrel. Never you."

Darrel grinned and walked away. It would have been unusual for him to get a ticket. He toed the line on every regulation and rule. That's why he did so well as a chemistry supervisor. It was his joy in life to do everything exactly and meticulously. The compulsive's compulsive.

Hank had always felt comfortable with compulsives. Did that make him one, too? Probably. Birds of a feather. Did he have more insight into this trait, then? Probably not. Too many times small deviations or diagnostic disagreements kept revolving in his mind late at night or even during vacations. Like an aberrant electric circuit, electrons never ceased spinning thoughts until he stopped what he was doing or got out of bed and wrote down the solution of the problem or a method to solve it.

Schmidt appeared later that morning, bustling about and requesting things in a loud voice. Apparently everything was an irritation. Schmidt had never shown this much agitation before. Things must not have gone well at the police station. Why? Don's report!

That's why Schmidt was at the station! Don's autopsy protocol had arrived and the chief wasted no time. He could see the chief now gently guiding with casual questions, asking Schmidt to explain the absence and probable disagreements in two autopsy findings.

Hank had been put through the same procedure a few times. It was pleasant and brief if you could substantiate your diagnoses. If you couldn't, the chief didn't change expression, but merely kept on probing about the basis for the interpretation. You quickly learned to keep your impressions separate from your diagnoses. Impressions weren't worth a bucket of warm spittle in court. A good deal of background information was unknown to the pathologist, so that gave the chief the upper hand.

Prosecuting attorneys changed with the political winds—the chief stayed on and on. He wasn't going to present anything to a green prosecutor until it was well laid-out.

The chief's method was to ask questions very diffidently, as though he didn't know the answer when he actually did. Chapter and verse had been checked out with another forensic pathologist or medical examiner. If you bluffed, he only nodded and slowly meandered about in his questions and backed you into a corner.

Hank could phrase the chief's approach. "Tell me about the two sets of fracture lines on the skull of Dr. Haims...Would you clue me in on what the microscope showed in the entrance wound? What chemical is it in the vitreous humor of the eyeball that is used to judge time of death?"

He could see Schmidt trying to use the obtuse terms and failing. "My opinion, based on reasonable medical certainty." That would be one of them. "My impression, based on my medical experience..." That would be another.

It wouldn't work. The chief would keep his granite face intact and pin the person resolutely. He had heard all the evasions and pompous phrases. One quick phone call eliminated any points of contention. Knowledge was disseminated continuously in workshops and seminars for police and ancillary personnel. Don's report had to agree with Hank's basic observations.

He signed out and went to the police station. The chief was gone but Monty was present.

"Dr. Markeley's report, please," demanded Hank.

Monty smiled. "Knew you'd be down." He handed Hank the report.

Hank quickly skimmed the findings, feeling satisfied.

"Thanks!" he said and left. Now he knew what the chemical was that smelled so strongly from the organs in the plastic sac. Returning to his office, he sat down with a pen again and began to sketch out his thoughts.

Suspects? Was the son still being traced? Had they ruled out Mrs. Haims? Yes, unless she had some quirky facets to her personality. Any other member of the Haims family who might have come home surreptitiously? Two other children were away at school; Jonathan, the son, would have been noticed if he came home. Did he?

Hank thought back to Schmidt's strange behavior. Aggression and desire to be head of the department was always the aim of any younger member. Expected everywhere. At least Hank wasn't pushed into the Arctic waters, put on an ice floe with food for a week like the Eskimos did with their discards—food being too scarce to feed a non-producer.

When does a doctor, like himself, lose his touch and become not only a non-producer but an embarrassment? Over the years, the lab had changed subtly. Why was there an undercurrent of animosity that sloshed around in brackish water? When did it begin? Did it begin with the appointment of Schmidt to the staff? Hank couldn't remember. Performance of a sloppy autopsy at an early hour before anyone could view the procedures. None of the others did that. Why did Schmidt? But he was biased against Schmidt and should be careful.

Then there was Sam. Cheerful, thoughtful, storytelling—Dr. Sam was everybody's friend. A suspect? Yes. Motive? Yes. Hidden hatred for injuring his child. What else? Patients meant money. Some people would do ghastly things for money. The amount of money was not necessarily relevant.

He had characterized Sam as easygoing and pleasant

without thinking. Was he? Everyone said so, therefore, a cynic would say the opposite.

Surgeons had to be able, by the very nature of their work, to set aside their feelings of empathy and cut flesh. Granted, it was inflicted to eliminate injuries or disease or cancer. The surgery was for the patient's overall benefit. Would Sam do away with Haims for his own personal benefit? Errant surgeons were known who lost their contact with reality and considered only the end result. Haims had been selected as chairman and president of various medical organizations. That spoke something and yet nothing for his standing in the medical community. Elections were a popular vote but all too often, no one wanted the position and a volunteer received the vote by default. Did Sam want these titles? As senior surgeon, they were now his for the asking.

Keith Gray. How much of a suspect? It was certainly possible. Keith ran in the early hours. Often odd hours. Compulsive running. He intimated that Darlene deteriorated mentally and physically for a time after the death of the only child. Darlene...hard to place her in a suspect category. Just the same, being a crack shot with a pistol and shooting competitively was an interesting facet. Typical of a father, wanting a boy and then teaching the girl the same activities. Motive and opportunity were present.

Patients of Haims's. A few lawsuits were pending. None appeared unusual. The larger the practice, the more vulnerable the physician. Span? No. Too subservient. Wimpy.

Cliff Evers? Cliff was used to hunting weapons and physical reaction to insult. He blamed Haims for the testicle infection that complicated his hernia/hydrocele surgery and caused the hormone and marriage problems. Someone said he had shadowed Haims for weeks. Just silently appeared wherever Haims was going until Haims complained to the police.

Hospital personnel were pretty much circumspect about Haims. They knew their jobs were all vulnerable if they displeased him. It was true that Haims had clout and anyone crossing Haims got the boot—including the administrator. Which meant Tim could have a motive? Possible versus probable. Tim kept his feelings controlled. He and his wife had worked too hard to achieve their positions and had good antennas for trouble. At the first sign of incompatibility, they would leave early on and keep moving until they found the right environment elsewhere.

Unless...unless Dr. Haims boxed them in somehow, with no alternatives. This would be unlikely. Haims's power stopped at St. Mary's.

Still to be explained was why Dr. Haims would chance his reputation by changing the pathological diagnoses. It would be found out eventually and was something impossible to conceal. Another hospital would want the patient's records, and all too often, the pathologist's report and microscopic slides were necessary to be reviewed. The differences in the diagnoses would be evident.

How would Haims cover up? Blame it on a computer mix-up? On a secretary? Blame the laboratory? Perhaps he simply became invulnerable in his own mind.

Why not? Hank tried to put himself into Haims's place and view the entire hospital as dependent on his wishes. It was a curiously powerful feeling if you pictured yourself as omnipotent.

In his mind, Hank began demanding special treatment in the form of being first on the surgery schedule, demanding certain operating rooms, certain types of music, certain nurses, anesthesiologists, radiologists, the X-ray doctors, special lockers... He demanded being president and on the board of trustees. All were given to him. Fact followed demand.

What would he do, as Haims, if challenged about his diagnosis of his patient's disease or abnormal tissue? Hank formed a reply and smiled, immensely pleased with himself in the reversed role as Haims. With no coaching, he could easily become The Total Emperor!

But it was reprehensible, childish behavior, abusing everyone under the guise of "the patient came first," and that it was all "being done for the patient's sake."

Still, changing a diagnoses required a twisted mind. Smoothing the way for payment was a lie. How did he get away with it so long? Had other physicians changed their diagnoses to fit payment patterns? To a reasonable degree, weren't many forced to shade their diagnoses? It would take a physician to ferret out the subtle differences. No lay auditor could do it with any confidence. He hadn't really checked other tissue diagnosis from surgery—just Haims's work. Hank got up and went to the medical record room.

"Let me see the last fifty surgical cases, please," he asked the clerk.

"Yes, Doctor." The little brown-eyed girl scurried away.

There was something satisfying about being the pathologist in a hospital. Years ago, when no other physician dared to inspect another physician's chart, the pathologist was allowed to see everything. The "watchdogs of the hospitals" were what they were known as then. The policemen. Now, with utilizations committees, critical care committees, tissue surgery committees, PRO and the like— well, much of the police action was placed on committee shoulders.

This was definitely for the better. Too much had depended upon the personality of the specific pathologist.

As humans are, some pathologists were too aggressive and others were too permissive. The aggressive ones lost their hospital appointments and were usually on borrowed time wherever they worked. The permissive ones were regarded as clerks or were ignored by the more astute physicians.

"What are you looking for, Doctor?"

The voice came from the supervisor of medical records. She was a good soul. Having once entered the convent and left, she sublimated by devoting her life to St. Mary's as she would have to the Order.

"Just checking pathological diagnoses in the surgical charts."

"Is something wrong?"

"I suppose not. Would like to see for myself, though."

The charts arrived and he was left alone. The supervisor had satisfied herself that there was no complaint about her work and had busied herself elsewhere. Still, it was an unusual request and it would be reported to the administrator.

The first five charts were satisfactory; no diagnosis had been changed. Then came the revelation with one chart. It re-appeared with another and then with another. These were not Dr. Haims's cases. He recognized fourteen diagnoses that had been modified—diseases substituted for normal tissue.

Hank felt creepy. He hadn't allowed for this. This was very bad. He sat stunned. Why hadn't he checked all the surgical charts before? He had found Haims's changes and quit. Why hadn't he been more thorough?

The supervisor came back. Her long, ankle-length skirt swishing. Fussing. Making conversation. Curious. There was no reason for her to go home—the hospital was her home.

"Isn't it too bad that Tim is leaving?" she said. "We'll

really miss him. He is so capable. And we love his wife so!" Her hands were clasped in front of her and her cross gleamed as it dangled over her chest.

Hank's thoughts stopped still. There it was! Tim was leaving! Tim knew something was foul and was getting out before the stink stuck to him. The meconium was not of his making. He had nothing to do with the manufacture of it, but he would be held accountable, just as he was held accountable everything that went on in the hospital.

Hank wondered how many other charts were involved and how long this had been going on. Did any of the other pathologists know about the changes? Someone had to have picked it up somehow—a question from a clerk; an original missing and a second copy request from the pathologist's files; insurance payment conflicts—all these were routine incidents.

The room became busy with many clerks who were wanting to work and he was occupying needed space. Only one clerk was on at night and she was kept fully occupied, typing up the patients' histories and physicals for the next day's surgeries.

He had better come back in the evening to check additional charts. Corky would be flying in soon. He'd better get to the airport.

Thirty

Corky was back. The children ran up and began showing him all the different gifts they had been given. Tape recorders, dolls, bow-and-arrow sets and many clothes. What would the world do without grandparents?

His father-in-law had even sent him a present: old copies of a financial newsletter. Obviously, he was worried about the future of his grandchildren, which meant Corky must have touched on the problems with his medical practice.

He smiled and thanked Corky, who knew his thoughts. Someday, perhaps financial magazines would interest him. Not now. If ever.

They sat and talked about her trip. After that, he explained what he had to do that evening. When she looked stricken, he promised it would be just two hours.

He left his family reluctantly. Only a cold, self-centered personality could pursue his own goals on the night of return of his family. A depressing thought, yet he *had* to clear himself as a suspect and the falsification of the charts had to be linked with Haims's murder. He was sure of it!

Hospital corridors were always eerie places at night. Partly because there was so much activity and conversation during the day that the same hallways, when quietly resting, seemed to take on strangely different, cold and forbidding personalities. So many unmarked doors opened from the long corridor into different areas of the hospital. Room use was constantly altered so often that no one could keep track of them.

Hank reflected on this as he punched the number on the security system to enter the hospital laboratory. The door buzzed and he noticed a light in the chief pathologist's room—his old room. A glance showed Dr. Schmidt working on some papers. He continued through the lab and greeted the night crew.

The usual stat problems were occurring. When three test orders arrive together, which test gets priority? No matter how the technologist chose, two of the three physicians would be unhappy with the slowness of their reports and complain to the pathologist and on occasion, to administration or to a committee.

Only a few years ago, a glucose test took two or more hours with the filtering and analysis. Now, if the attending physician had to wait more than a few minutes, he became angry. No matter how fast the tests were performed, expectations exceeded the fastest performance—all because very meager hands-on laboratory testing was taught in the medical schools. Of course, a good part of the reason was that no laboratory could afford to turn a medical students loose onto a $150,000 chemistry instrument/computer without offering extensive training.

After a brief conversation with the busy techs, Hank proceeded up to the medical records unit. Sandy, the librarian whom he knew, was busy alternating her typing with pauses of listening through her ear phones. She spied him and stopped.

"Listen to this word, will you, Doctor? I'm not sure I can understand what is being said. Retro...something?"

Hank put on the earphones.

"Retroperitoneal and periaortic," he answered.

"Thank you. It comes through as a mumble sometimes. What would you like?"

"Sandy, I'd like the surgical charts for the past three months. How hard would it be to pull those?"

"You're kidding! Say you're joking!" Sandy looked aghast.

"No, no," said Hank quickly. "I mean just the surgical charts involving tissue removed in the operating room."

"Wow! That's better! Sure. Take ten minutes. Okay?" She was as good as her word. She returned triumphant.

"How come so quick?"

"Tissue surgery committee meets Thursday. They had to be pulled for review—three months' worth."

"I thought they met monthly?"

"They do, but for some reason, joint commission is coming through to accredit the hospital and they specifically want to review certain surgicals and confirm reasons for the surgery."

"Hmm. Thanks. I'll sit back there out of the way."

Hank moved the mass of charts to the back wall next to a desk. He took a clean sheet of paper from the drawer and began taking notes.

After an hour, he had finished almost all the charts. With a sinking feeling, he realized that the pattern was not limited to Dr. Haims.

"I'm leaving!" shouted Sandy. "Turn off the lights when you leave, please."

"Where do you want the charts placed?" His voice echoed.

"Right there is fine. They'll retrieve them for the committee easy enough. Good night."

Without another human present, the room seemed different. The quietness was unnatural. The continuous rush of air through the ducts seemed louder than normal. Creaking doors and muffled footsteps permeated the entire area. It had to be his imagination. He was concentrating so deeply, he jumped when a hand touched his shoulder.

"Still at it?" It was Keith.

"Why, yes. What are you doing here? You have early surgeries tomorrow."

"Oh, emergency surgeries. Husband stabbed wife so the wife shot husband. Fun and games for several hours."

"Who operated?"

"Two teams of surgeons. Plenty to do for all of them. Saw a light back here and saw you bending over the charts. Committee work or still personal investigative work?"

"Something of both." Hank felt reluctant to be specific.

"Well, enjoy yourself. Nothing duller than reviewing charts."

Keith left, but not before his inquisitive eyes had taken in the fact that Hank was making a list.

Keith could easily surmise what Hank was after, since he already knew the problem about discrepancies in diagnoses. Finishing up quickly, he left the charts in the corner where he was working and left the back door of the hospital.

It was an abnormally dark night with continuing strange sounds that had to be his imagination again, working overtime.

For safety's sake, he had parked his car under the street lamp since the episode of the beating. He was ready for any quick movements anywhere.

As he turned the street corner to enter the parking lot, there was a muffled sound behind him and before he could turn, he felt a terrible pain in back of his head. As he slipped into unconsciousness, he could feel someone's labored breathing over his face.

That was all.

Thirty-one

When he woke up he knew he was in the emergency room. He had performed too many procedures in every room not to recognize each one well. White on white everywhere except his brain.

He slipped back into semiconsciousness. The back of his head hurt and his mind was groggy but no one came to assist him. He groaned and called out.

A nurse he knew looked in and said, rather abruptly, "We'll see you in a minute. We're real busy right now." Her face was severe.

He waited. The pain was still there. He tried to get up. He was dizzy. It took some doing but slowly he managed.

No one came in to assist.

Wait a moment. What was that smell? Alcohol. Why were they using so much? The smell was overpowering! It penetrated his nostrils, almost choking him. It took awhile for him to realize that it wasn't the room. It was him!

Without thinking, he staggered off the bed, out of the room and down the hall. Still, no one came to his assistance. The nurse, who came into the room before, was seated, writing on a chart. She was trying to ignore him but he knew she saw him. She was not that busy—his practiced eye knew that.

"I'm heading out. My head hurts. What happened?"

She looked up at Hank silently and without sympathy. That was unusual for her. The E.R. doctor bustled by on his way to a room. A child was crying. Someone was moaning.

"Hi, Doctor. Had a few too many, did you?"

"No. I was leaving the hospital and got hit in back of the head."

The emergency room doctor hesitated. "Right! The ground is awful hard these days."

"No. I mean it. I was struck from behind."

"Well, maybe you've forgotten. The whiskey bottle was pretty well drained dry." His voice dropped low. "Don't worry. We'll keep it quiet. No records will be kept."

"No, really...I mean it. I wasn't drinking."

The E.R. doctor and nurse exchanged glances. Should they believe him? They knew from hospital gossip he had been demoted from department head and drew definite conclusions. Drunks who denied they had been drinking were all too common.

"Well, see you tomorrow, then!" The E.R. people had too much to do that required immediate attention. No matter who it was, a drunk was a drunk. Hank left. Why explain?

Where did he park his car? Normally, he had difficulty remembering where he parked his car. Now, it was doubly difficult. Finally, he found it.

The driver's seat was ripped open. Whiskey bottles were strewn on the front floor. Little single-ounce bottles. The interior stank of liquor. For some reason, he sat and didn't start the car. Something wasn't right. He lifted the hood. Nothing. Then he checked the outside. A tire was flat.

Corky would be asleep now. No use getting her up.

Avoiding the emergency room, he walked around the outside of the hospital to the laboratory. If only he didn't smell of sour whiskey! It reeked!

As he was calling a cab, a tech stuck her neck into the room, saw him and grimaced. Naturally, with his luck, it would be Hazel, the "granola-clean" type who abhorred liquor, tobacco and any of life's sinful and base pleasures. And just as naturally, she would relate his appearance all over the hospital.

Hank ignored what she was saying. He felt worse than before. He held his head in his hands. Air. He needed air. Walking quickly, he left the lab and stood outside on the corner, partly hidden by the dogwood trees. The cab seemed to take hours but finally arrived. Hank waved him down.

The cab driver was wary at first because of the way he weaved as he walked, but changed his mind after he recognized Hank. Then he became overly courteous and energetically launched into praising him for calling a cab and not driving.

The cabbie's upbeat, bright conversation lasted until his destination. It wasn't until he reached into his pocket to pay the cab that he noticed that the sheet of paper was gone. All the suspicious surgical pathology numbers he had copied down from the medical charts were gone. His wallet was there. Three hours of work for nothing. He'd have to do it all over again.

"It's okay, Doc. You can pay me tomorrow. Don't worry about it."

"No. No. Here it is." Hank added a generous tip.

The cabby left after a cheerful "Call me anytime."

He went into the house and went to the bathroom. His face was puffy. He looked terrible. As he undressed, Corky woke up and greeted him with a worried expression. "You're terribly late and you smell bad. Is that alcohol? Where did you go? Who did you meet?"

"Can't convince anyone in E.R. that I was hit on the head near the hospital parking lot. I'll tell the chief in the morning—an ordinary cop won't believe it."

She sat upright and shook her head to grasp what he was saying. "Really...if you decided to have a few drinks, it's all right. You can tell me... I half-expected it."

"Haven't had a drop."

"Let me smell your breath."

"It's there, too. Whoever did it, also spilled some in my mouth."

"Hmmm." Corky looked at him speculatively.

"They didn't believe me in the E.R., either."

"You went there?"

"I found myself there. Under avoided gazes—and what passes for professional care—only no one sympathizes with a drunk in E.R. They see too many godawful accidents due to drinking."

"Then you were drunk."

"No!" Hank shook his head too vigorously and ascended the stairs. "I'll talk to you in the morning. My head still hurts."

"Well, I should think it should," said Corky. "How

much did you drink…or spill…or whatever you call it?"

Wordlessly, Hank went to the other side of the bed and fell on it and was immediately asleep.

She undressed him and covered him up like one of the children. She was wide awake now and sat for a long time on the bed, thinking about what was happening. Hank was doing bizarre things and acting strangely.

Where had he really been tonight? And why? Her dad had his informants in business. Now she had to rely on hers.

Thirty-two

"Are you ready to talk about it?" It was the next morning and a worried Corky was watching him carefully. The children were still asleep.

"Right after breakfast. Coffee, please." Hank felt groggy and very tired. He felt the back of his head. Still there. A large lump was now present.

After the second cup, he began to describe what he had done and what happened. Corky's wariness changed from sympathy to fear. That's the reaction he expected. It was always this way when she couldn't be involved personally in a situation. She listened carefully and made no comment.

Corky drove him to the laboratory. Dr. Schmidt was already there, looking very officious, and nodded curtly to him while he dialed the telephone.

"Dr. Havermann wanted to meet with you as soon as you came in."

"He's the chief of staff right now, isn't he?"

"That's right!" Schmidt beamed pompously.

Hank went behind the desk, put his feet up and picked up some reading material. The headache made it difficult to concentrate. When Dr. Havermann came into the room, Hank glanced up questioningly. Schmidt followed behind and closed the door behind him.

"Why the closed door?" Hank asked. "Poison is safer and quieter and certain toxins will never be found—or do you need help in their selection?"

Dr. Havermann was known for not having a modicum of humor. "Your behavior is not a joking matter, Doctor."

Hank knew Havermann disliked pathologists—all pathologists. Prior to attending medical school, Havermann had worked in a laboratory and had been subjected to ridicule by a pathologist who had been difficult to please. He never forgave the pathologist and hated all laboratorians from that day on.

"My behavior is always a joke...as is life on this planet," said Hank as he looked at the tips of his shoes. They needed polishing.

Dr. Havermann drew himself up to his full height and glared. Even his glasses gleamed with dislike. "Getting drunk and disoriented while on duty constitutes moral turpitude and is grounds for dismissal from the medical staff. I hope you will take that seriously."

"It makes us look so bad in the laboratory!" added Schmidt sanctimoniously, almost wringing his hands.

"Worse is sloppy work. Chief Enzer explain that to

you?" Hank looked at Schmidt directly.

Schmidt flushed and bit his mustache.

Dr. Havermann looked at them both. "I'm sorry, but he will have to be reported to the ethics committee, Dr. Schmidt." Dr. Havermann tried to appear reluctant, but his eyes were dancing with pleasure.

Hank smiled at Havermann. "The ethics committee will refer it to the executive committee, who will then return it to the ethics committee for corroboration, who will then pass the buck to the Physician's Recovery Network. The latter committee deals with chemical addictions of all sorts. I know. I'm chairman."

"So you expect to have this whitewashed and swept under the carpet?"

"Since you don't know the facts, it won't get past the first committee."

"What do you have to say in your defense?" asked Dr. Havermann sternly, trying to recapture the official nature of the meeting.

Hank put down the reading material. "The last word is 'arschloch,' which is a euphonious term indicating an object from which noxious smells and waste products emanate. I feel badly, insulting such a useful part of the anatomy by applying it to you."

Hank looked at Schmidt. "And you. Leave the door open, please. But leave." Hank let the papers lie in his lap as he continued to stare through the tips of his shoes.

It was Havermann's next statement that made Hank wish he had booted them both. Hard. "I'll talk to the administrator right away." Dr. Havermann spoke to Schmidt outside the door so Hank could hear. "He'll know the correct procedure to follow."

Damn! Didn't they ever let up stop appointing themselves as keepers of the morals—for everyone else? Both would have fit into the Middle Ages perfectly!

He lifted a sheet of paper from his desk. It was a report that had been opened by one of the other pathologists, initialed without comment and sent to him, since it was a bone marrow interpretation Hank had performed.

The hematologist said that the polyclonal gammopathy was just that and nothing else. Hank had read it as polyclonal gammopathy also, but more seriously suggested the cells were going to eventuate into multiple myeloma, a bone cancer caused by excessive myeloma cells. Hank had based his opinion on other factors besides increased numbers of plasma cells. The seventy-eight-year-old patient was getting more anemic every month and disturbingly enough, had no other symptoms or diseases such as lupus, arthritis, or auto-immune factors to account for the gammopathy.

Was he wrong? Kappa and lambda light chains would tell. Usually a myeloma showed exclusively one type of chain, whereas a simple plasmacytosis or reaction to a chronic disease showed both. He could stain the bone marrow smears and ask the clinician to check the patient's urine for light chains.

Hank called the chief hematology tech and asked for the stains to be performed. He called the patient's doctor and discussed the case. A sedimentation rate of 90mm an hour was very high and occurred only with an active inflammatory process—which the clinician denied that the patient had—or with malignancy.

"What are you doing here?" Looking aghast was Ed Wilkins, the associate pathologist, in his doorway.

"Working or what passes for work."

"You're supposed to be doing the anatomic surgery! We switched services this morning!" Ed Wilkins was angry and unsmiling. Usually polite, he was either feeling out of sorts this morning, or worse, felt Hank would be no longer a viable consideration as a colleague, much less as the department head.

"Forgot to look at the schedule, Ed. Is it smelling that bad?"

"Is what smelling bad? I don't smell anything. Is bacteriology cooking agar again?"

"Vultures and dead fish! Never mind. I'll handle the anatomic and the frozens."

"Well, they're calling for a pathologist in surgery right now! You know I hate frozen sections!" Ed justified his agitation with righteous indignation.

"That's the first time you admitted it—I suspected such when you always took your vacation during this time of service. Time me! Thirty seconds. I'll be in surgery. Quick enough?"

The reprimand was flung with a grin—no one could take Ed's concerns seriously. His wife, nicknamed "the general," ran his life and even mowed the lawn for him. Ed was very good after studying a problem slide for days, detailing the diagnoses with care, describing the trees in the forest, the rocks and the streams and redoing it after checking it with the university pathologists. Then he added references for a final florish. Clinicians groaned when they were informed that Ed was investigating the case.

"Dr. Feinstein wants the lymph node checked for Hodgkin's disease." The nurse handed him a basin containing a small piece of tissue covered with wet gauze.

Hank looked at the tissue and called the surgical suite over the intercom. "Can't check for lymphoma on a frozen section, Doctor. Sorry," he said.

"If you can't give me what I need, forget it!" came the exasperated reply over the loudspeaker.

He heard the surgeon grumble loudly to the surgical

personnel before he shut off the communication: "When you need help, those pathologists never come through! It's a waste of time asking them to look at anything. I don't know why I bother!"

Nasty. But then, Feinstein was the surgeon for the Hyco Corporation and all the workers at the plant were contracted to his clinic. If the workers wanted to choose their own surgeon, then the plant insurance would only cover a small percentage of the cost.

Hank returned to his room. A note was plastered on the desk lamp from administration. "At your convenience, please call the associate hospital administrator."

One more blast from administration was too much! Could he control his temper?

Thirty-three

George Temple was quite different than Tim in personality, almost opposite—open, relaxed, and straightfor-
ward in his responses. It had been fun to chat with him
before. What about this time?

"Hi, George. What's up? Checking into hospital drunks
these days?" said Hank. "Sounds like a come-down for
you."

George's blue eyes winced—his pleasant face became
troubled. "Oh, come on, Hank," he said, "Tim asked me to
check into this and defuse the situation. There must be an
easy explanation. Dr. Havermann came storming into the
office this morning and wants you fired or else he's going

to go before the medical staff and have you voted out. What's it all about? You're not a drinker." The same George. Open. Honest, as always.

"Are you sure? Could be one of those closet types, you know," suggested Hank.

George looked bewildered. "All I know is, you've been having one hell of a time! Haims dug at you and got you demoted; Span comes in for a copy of the staff bylaws and gets a committee together to pound on you; you get attacked in our parking lot and now—this drinking business! What's going on?"

"You've just summarized it, George."

"There must be more. Do you know who it is? They really want you off the staff and practicing elsewhere!"

"Right," agreed Hank.

"Yeah. I suppose anything is possible, but Dr. Havermann is always bitching like an old woman about someone, so you're not alone. He and Dr. Haims were bitter about each other."

"I thought they were related?" said Hank, surprised.

"They are, I guess. But we couldn't put them both on the same committee, for example."

"Haims had Span—who made up for it."

"Yes," said George with a grimace. "We all know Dr. Span."

"Then you'll believe me if I tell you I got hit on the head, had whiskey poured in my mouth and on my clothes?"

"If you say so, I believe it. I'll report it that way."

Hank felt surprise at the warmth of the response. "George! You're a jewel in a mudhole. A cowboy expression."

"You've got the advantage on me—I'm not a horse person," said George. "After you were attacked the first time, we put in two more poles with those big sodium lights."

"Well, thanks. That was thoughtful."

"We figured if it happened to you, it could happen to anyone. Were you hurt? Did you tell the police?"

"The first time I told the police. The second time, I had something that someone wanted and it wasn't money. Is that all you wanted to talk to me about?

George blinked and nodded.

"How's the banjo?" asked Hank.

"I knew you'd bring up the banjo." George laughed. "I only wondered how you would work it into the conversation this time."

Hank's eyes crinkled. "Been scientifically proven that banjo enthusiasts are a black blot on civilized musical societies. Unstable character trait."

"When you start that, I know it's time for me to sign off," said George, looking at his desk. "Auxiliary meets in five minutes. Seriously, who do you think is after you? With Dr. Haims's murder, I'm ready to believe anything."

"I've a definite suspicion about the beating in the parking lot—it came too fast after an argument. This last, with the alcohol, was deliberate and carefully done."

"Well, you've got a friend here whenever you need help."

"Thanks, George. You're a great guy, even though you play the banjo."

"See you," laughed George, as he headed for another of his multiple hospital meetings.

When Hank returned to his office, a call came in from the School of Nursing. They needed a lecture on fluid balance right away. That afternoon?

Hank groaned. Someone else had canceled at the last minute and they knew he never refused. Lectures forced him to brush up on fundamentals. It took thirty minutes for him to review his previous lecture notes and he signed out to the other pathologists.

At the school, he found himself being stared at by twenty-odd student nurses who ranged in age from late teens to mid-fifties.

The talk went well. The questions were pertinent and sensible. A question about the difference between osmolarity and osmolality took him back in time when he was a student and had accepted the two words as similarities. The associate dean had corrected him. One didn't forget things like that. Part of the learning process. Afterward, when he was packing up the projector to leave, a student came up to him, timidly.

"Doctor," she said. "I saw something I should tell you about."

"Yes?"

"The other night in the parking lot when I got off-duty, I saw someone lying on the ground next to a car and a large figure was standing over him and pouring something on him. I stopped and asked if I could help, and the person bending over said, 'No! No! Scram! It's my cousin—he's drunk. I'll take care of it.' He had his back to me and was so nasty about it that I left. It wasn't until just now that someone whispered that you were in the E.R., smelling of whiskey and complaining of being hit on the head."

"Could you remember the figure or what he was wearing?"

"Not really, but he was large and wearing a coat with a fur collar."

"Tall, short?"

"I'm sorry. It was dark at night. Large, though."

"Large in the sense of fat?"

"Yes. More in the sense of fat."

"Thanks. That helps."

The student nurse walked away.

Thirty-four

In the hospital, Hank found Keith in the anesthesiology department, scheduling for the different operating rooms.

"Looking for anesthesia?" asked Keith. "You're in the right place."

"No, thanks. Keith, do you remember the other night when I was working in the medical records room?"

"Sure. Big night in out-patient surgery. Chaos!"

"Who were the doctors there?"

"Seemed like they were all there. Let me see: Himmelbaker, Martins, England, Koerner...Why, even a pathologist was there—Schmidt!"

"Surgeons?"

"Why, Heuksingwald, Stancowitz, Spitzer, Thornton..."

"Any of them leave early?"

"Most were through by the time I left. A few stayed and talked to the parents and family. Why?"

"I was hit on the head and sloshed over with whiskey right after you left."

"I heard about that! Rumor had it that...are you all right now? This small town is getting to be a rough place!" Keith's concern appeared genuine. Was it?

"Yep," said Hank. "Couldn't convince E.R. I wasn't drunk. Also a problem now with Dr. Havermann, who felt it constituted moral turpitude."

"Self-righteous jerk."

"I gathered from his indignation."

"What's he have to do with you?"

"He's president of the medical staff now."

"Right! I forgot." Keith smiled. "Or repressed it."

"Thanks."

"Anything else I can do—let me know. I'm sure sorry." Keith was back into his scheduling.

Who else should he check with? Large, bulky figure. Or was it the angle of his viewing? A body bending over you would naturally feel larger than normal.

The fur collar! Who would know about which doctors wore fur collars? Yesterday. Operating room? No. The doctor's lounge was separate. The E.R. nursing supervisor. Jan Lewis. She would know. Jan never missed a thing, including loose threads and untied shoelaces.

Fur collars. They were not in vogue. He was certain only a few physicians would wear them. Who? He never noticed.

Jan was talking to a nurse. He waited. When she looked

up and saw Hank, she terminated her conversation. "Hello, stranger. Nice to see you sober. Are you lost? Or are you looking for AA?"

"Need your help." Hank sat in the chair next to her desk.

"So do a lot of other people."

"But I really do! Question: Which of the doctors wears a coat with a fur collar or has fur on his lapel?"

"That's easy. Your partner, Dr. Schmidt, for one. Dr. French, Dr. Olman did, but doesn't anymore, Dr. Sam—Why, are you planning to upgrade your wardrobe?" Hank got up to leave, but Jan had other ideas. "Why did you want to know?" Her eyes bored into him.

"It's important."

Jan's eyes became glazed. She thought out loud. "So the guy who bopped you was wearing a coat with a fur collar..."

"I didn't say that."

"No."

"You and Keith in anesthesiologist do all kinds of deducing!" said Hank. "How do you know I wasn't potted?"

Jan snorted with laughter. "You're not the type."

"Why not?" Hank was humbled.

"Just impossible. That's all."

"Now you make me sound like a cold robot. My Corky's words."

"Really? She said that now?" Jan's eyes twinkled. "Cold robot, eh? We agree and I've only known you for nine or ten years. Snap judgment on our part."

"Well, thanks, for your confidence."

"That's not all. You'll find him."

"How can you be so sure?" Hank asked, surprised.

Jan looked at him quietly. "You wear things down until they're resolved. You are known for your persistence around here, you know. Quiet, gentlemanly, but persistent."

"Thanks...I guess." Interesting how others saw you.

He headed for the Rodeo Grounds. Corky and the children were there. The Grounds were dusty and horses were everywhere—being groomed, saddled, unsaddled, trained or simply ridden.

"Doc!" The voice was shouting after him.

It was Cliff Evers, dressed in his usual jeans, shirt and rolled cowboy hat. He ambled up with a loose, rolling motion. "You know that cutting doctor that got murdered?"

"Yes."

"They keep trying to stick me with doin' him in."

"Oh?"

"Yep. Lucky they can't find bleeding hemorrhoids in the snow."

"It's their job. Anybody who had a beef against Dr. Haims is checked out." Hank felt the pomposity of his statement.

"Don't matter. Maybe I'd like to have, after what he done to me, but I didn't! Just wanted you to know, that's all."

Cliff had singled him out to tell him something important. He knew something about the murder but some sort of code he had learned prevented him from squealing or ratting.

A misguided sense of honor. He'd tell another cowboy or rancher because they belonged. Hank didn't. Nothing personal.

"How do you like the doctor I sent you to see?" asked Hank.

"I think she's helped me already. I trust her—she's a lot better than the other guy the cutting doctor sent me to."

Cliff made a low wave of his hand and walked away with a self-confident roll to his body which started from his boots on up. Hank observed that Cliff's mental depression was gone and made a note to send Dr. Jane a large box of M & M's—her favorite.

Hank met Corky, who was riding and tried to discuss his conversation with Cliff and his suspicions.

She was too happy to care—once she was on a horse, she was a different person. He saddled up and they rode together until dark, trying to avoid those who would ask questions about Haims's death.

The three children were collected—they had been roaming all over with a borrowed Shetland pony. The children's problems were enough for her to handle. The previous night had eliminated a great deal of her reserve.

Thirty-five

The telephone set off one of its urgent type of rings. "Hank! Hank! It's me, Louie," the excited voice said.

Hank held the telephone receiver to his ear, glanced at the alarm clock by habit and woke up immediately. Lou Gavins had never called him at home before.

"Yo, Louie! Something's wrong?" Was it one of their horses?

"I just called 911. We've got a dead man here—hanging from the rafters in the horse stall."

"Who is it, Lou?"

"It looks like…Cliff! My Gawd, I hope it's not, but—"

"You didn't cut him down, did you?"

"No. I could tell there was no hope of savin' im. His face is all colors and his tongue…Gawd, it's awful. I called 911 and then I thought of you, you being in the autopsy business and all that…you would know about this kind of thing."

"Leave him alone, Lou. Don't touch anything. The medics will know to back off. Don't let anyone near the stall."

"Okay, Doc. I won't.

The drive to the Rodeo Grounds took ten minutes. The police chief was already there, the entrance was blocked and Hank had to park his car and walk in through a hole in the fence. Yellow tape surrounded the area.

"Hi, Doc. You here to see the body?" asked the sergeant, who recognized him and the reason he had come.

"Yes." Hank put the plastic bags over his shoes and walked into the horse stall. The cowboy's face was a blotched tan color and his tongue protruded.

"What do you think?" The police chief was at his shoulder.

"Needs a post," said Hank. "Who do you want to do it? Not me, I suppose. Dr. Markeley?"

Chief Enzer hesitated. The expense of Dr. Markeley he could justify once. Twice so soon would put his relations with the coroner on a very touchy basis.

"If you did it, how soon would you begin?" he asked.

"Right now."

"Good! I was hoping you would say that. We'll watch." Chief Enzer blinked his approval.

"Get him to the morgue with a signed permit. I'll be waiting."

Fifteen minutes later, by the time the body arrived, Hank had set up the table, spread out the cutting implements and empty receptacle jars, some of which contained formalin, and had two rolls of film ready. Four police officers arrived with the chief. One had a camera.

Hank placed the autopsy number on the clothed body and began taking pictures. He waited for the policeman to take a back-up photo each time.

Satisfied, he began removing the clothes, leaving the rope around the neck intact, constantly looking for any-thing else that was unusual.

Then he began his external examination of the body and finally cut the rope in back of the neck, avoiding the knot. The marks of the ligature on the neck were faint, so he moved the light closer for better pictures. He began a meticulous search of the skin, started with the head and scalp and extending downward.

"Found it!" he said to the police chief. "The needle mark."

"Cliff...a drug addict?" The chief looked puzzled.

"No." Hank began taking close-ups pictures of the needle tract. "Only one needle mark I can see in an extraordinary place. The ones in the antecubital veins—the veins on the inside of the lower arm—we did here, when we took his blood for testing. This one, you'll agree, is very different." Hank incised the surface and the wall of the organ, placing samples into a special container.

"So...what do you think?" Chief Enzer was peering at the needle mark as though willing it to speak.

"Murder. I was suspicious when the color of his face was wrong for a hanging. Also, there aren't any Tardieu spots—little pinpoint hemorrhages—on the sclera. These always occur from the pressure of the blood in the neck blood vessels. I'll wager the hyoid bone in the neck, which usually gets fractured in a real hanging, is intact."

"What are you doing now?" asked the chief.

"Cutting wide around the needle tract so tissue analysis

can be performed. Next, I'll get some blood and urine for toxi- screen. The chemical smell is definite again."

Hank continued with the remainder of the autopsy, leaving the most important aspects—the brain and the neck—until last.

There were firm fibrous adhesions in both inguinal areas where the hernia surgery was performed. The bladder was full. He removed 50 ccs with a syringe and placed it in a sterile container. Some thick yellow residual material was at the base of the bladder. He removed the prostate and both testes. One was atrophic; the other was soft and had a few yellow-green areas throughout—partially healed. A mixed bacterial population probably with Pseudomonas organisms likely. He took a sterile swab and cultured the material aerobically and also anaerobically.

Having finished the chest, abdomen and pelvis, he turned to the neck. Sure enough! The hyoid and thyroid bones were intact and no hemorrhage was present in the strap muscles in the neck. This confirmed it. Cliff had been strung up after he had been killed.

Dr. Schmidt quietly walked in. Although less arrogant in demeanor than before, he began leaning over Hank's shoulder, as though justifying his presence by explaining what Hank was doing to the other police officers. Schmidt avoided looking at the chief.

"Augh!" Schmidt screamed as blood spurted into his face. "Aught!"

"Sorry. Slipped," said Hank, appearing contrite.

Schmidt ran over to the sink to wash off the blood covering his face. "Damn you, Whipple! You did that on purpose!" he shouted.

Hank was laconic. "Could have been worse...it was only a lung I was putting in the bag when it could have been the two thousand-gram liver!"

Schmidt continued his washing until he was satisfied everything was clean. The police chief watched Schmidt with interest.

"Cliff was only a carrier for AIDS—no symptoms as yet?" asked someone in the group.

Hank, startled, looked up from the autopsy and at the policemen.

Schmidt's eyes widened. He looked from one to the other and began to sputter. Then he abruptly left the room.

"Dr. Schmidt absolutely panics with any mention of AIDS. I can tell you for sure, he's out there getting a computer printout on all of Cliff's lab work. Shame!" said Hank.

A policeman laughed. "You won't take it personal if I don't get too near you, Doc? A little organ-sloshin' goes a long way!"

"Actually, we're mostly through with the essential findings, except for one last job," said Hank.

"Call me in the morning then?" asked Chief Enzer. The policemen looked relieved at taking leave. They knew the next procedure Hank was to perform.

"Preliminaries," Hank replied. "The tissue analyses will take time—unless I find a significant amount of that chemical available in the organ."

Hank carefully triple-bagged the tissue containing the needle mark and eliminating as much air as possible. Then he took large pieces of both lungs, liver, kidney, the gall bladder and tied off the esophageal and duodenal ends of the stomach. An hour had elapsed since he had drained a cc of the vitreous humor—the fluid which filled an eyeball. In another hour, he would take a second sample from the other eye.

He waited until the chief and his officers left before he sliced the scalp from mastoid to mastoid and folded back the skin, forward and backward. From experience, he knew the policemen could take a lot, except when it came to the noise of the saw cutting through the cranium.

Hank grunted with what he saw as he reflected back the scalp. He reached for the camera and took pictures of the fracture lines. They were somewhat similar to those he saw on Haims's skull.

Next was sawing open the top of the cranium, leaving a notch in the front, so replacement later wouldn't cause the cranium to twist sideways under the head.

How could he perform an autopsy on a friend?

By subterfuge. By fooling his eyes—whenever he performed an autopsy, he routinely covered the face with a cloth. It worked. The person became just another body…a body that would yield the necessary clues which caused death.

Sure enough, abundant blood was covering the leptomeninges—the inner two layers of the thin membranes covering the brain. He took pictures and gently removed the clots. It was quite a bash—the brain was cut by the multiple fragments of bone.

Overkill. Skull fracture, injection and hanging. The killer was going beyond not taking any chances—which meant Cliff not only knew the killer, but posed a threat. A threat to what? It could only be knowledge. Hank reached for the camera again.

The autopsy over, Hank went to his office and wrote out the preliminary findings on Cliff's death. It was well past 2 A.M. when he returned home.

Thirty-six

The next morning, he picked up the typed report and took it to the police station. He had become familiar enough for the sergeant to merely wave him to the back. The chief's door was open.

"You know there are similarities in the methods of murder of Dr. Haims and Cliff?"

"It would seem."

"Cliff disliked Haims very much."

"Checked it out long ago." The chief's eyes were unblinking.

Hank hesitated. "I always feel stupid when I tell you things you already know."

"Hmmm. You said it. I didn't."

Hank sighed. "You probably also know about having whiskey poured on me the other night. Any ideas?"

"Probably related to the fur collar bit you've been inquiring about."

"Good God! Isn't there anything you don't know about that goes on in this town?" Hank laughed.

"My town." The words expressed definite ownership. Like a car or home. It was his manner of speaking that caused Hank to reflect, "You've got somebody stashed at E.R. in the hospital."

"Can't deny or confirm." The chief smiled slightly.

"Also all taxis. Airport too, I'll bet. Bars. Restaurants. Anything suspicious or out of the ordinary gets called to you." Hank stated it as a fact.

"You're after my job, Doctor! I'm going to have to watch it." The chief had edged down the hall as they spoke.

He commenced whistling as he picked up a cup of coffee from the trustee, stopped a moment, looked back at Hank without expression and went into his office.

When Hank returned to the lab, the secretary told him Hermy, their supervisor, needed to talk to him. She had another problem about quality control using Hempter reagents. He wrote a memo, enclosed copies of their worksheets and put them in the mail.

"Dr. Sager sent us some more flowers for the benign diagnosis on his golfing partner. The one with Infectious Mono. They're very pretty!" said Hermy.

"I remember," Hank said as he visualized Sam Sager swinging a golf club. A natural mannerism of his was to swing—at the end of a joke. The punch line seemed to demand a swing...of a club.

Interruption. Steve Blodgett was glaring at him from the doorway.

"What do you want, Blodgett?"

"How much?" Blodgett's mouth was grim.

"How much what?"

"What do you want to bug off? Your memos to Minneapolis have caused all kinds of trouble for us. We're a respectable, multimillion-dollar firm and we're about to sue you, unless you quit telling everyone our chemicals are inferior!"

"Did they tell you it was all documented that they are inferior? This week we tried six different lots of your reagents and they all gave different results. We've got this documented as well and additional memos have been sent to the administrator here and to Minnesota."

Blodgett said, "You're one of the few who give us this kind of trouble. For your information, I've already replaced the chemicals you're talking about. Antibody tests are extremely difficult to make perfectly."

"And your company is probably the most imperfect in the field." Hank turned back to his work.

"Okay," Blodgett snarled. "We know how to play hard ball with wise guys. You only work here, remember. You seem to need a bigger sample."

A bigger sample. The words spun in the air. Idle threats from a salesman concerned about losing a commission? How much of a commission?

He got up but Blodgett had disappeared. Hank went into every department, searching. "Carol," he said when he found the executive secretary, "how large is the monthly statement from Hempster?"

"Easily twelve thousand," she replied without hesitation. "Some months higher, depending on what instruments are on lease."

"Then…we're talking about $750,000 for a five-year contract?"

"Ummm. More, if you add in the instruments. They

have other hospitals in St. Mary's Order—so you can multiply—"

"Yes. The administrator informed me. Thanks."

Hank went back to his desk and began thinking about Blodgett. The stakes were high. Five-year contracts with all five hospitals times almost a million dollars each...no wonder Blodgett was furious and willing to threaten, bribe...

He needed a breather and thought of the Roundup Grounds, even though he'd still be questioned by everyone about Cliff.

Hank clipped on his beeper, got into his car and drove off. Immediately, he noticed a car following. Blodgett? No. He took several different turns, thought he'd lost it, but found it stayed tight behind him—almost bumper to bumper. He was tired of being pushed. Two blocks from the Grounds, he stopped the car and got out.

"Why are you following me?"

With an evil grin, the other driver got out. Black jacket. Heavy boots. Sleek brown hair covering part of his face. He was slipping something over his knuckles— anticipating a fight.

"Because you learn slow, I hear!" said the man, walking up close. Without any preliminaries, he suddenly swung.

The blow came from the left—just like—it *was* the same one who attacked him in the parking lot! Hank just had time to twist away but caught the edge of the swing. Even so, it hurt. But the follow-up kick into his groin hurt more.

This was a brawler who relished beating up people. Hank had foolishly waited until they were in a remote area of the city—few cars passed in the open acreages near the Grounds.

All Hank could do is dodge and watch the arms and feet.

If it was a matter of time that he got beat up, then at least he'd give as good as he could.

Hank took three fast blows and twisted away, gasping for breath. The figure moved toward him, confident. He cocked his arm as he drew it back. The metal over his knuckles gleamed in the sunlight.

Hank waited until the last moment and leaned out. At the same time, he allowed part of the man's momentum to swing into his own fist. It smashed, hard, full force, into his face.

Using the surprise factor and hesitation, Hank quickly slipped behind him, threw his arm around his neck, bent backward and dropped him onto the ground. Before he could recover, Hank placed his foot over the larynx.

"Move and you stop breathing! I'll break your neck!"

Ignoring the threat, the figure twisted and tried to snap up. Hank jammed his foot down hard, using all his weight. Grabbing his throat, the figure rolled up and bent down on his knees. The fight seemed to be over. With dirty fighting, it was never over. Hank remained wary.

Without warning, the figure lunged at his legs and tried to bring Hank down, but was too weakened from gasping for breath. The fight was over.

"Hold it right there!" commanded a voice. Policeman. Squad car.

"How long were you here?" Hank asked.

"Just now," he said, quickly flipping the assailant's hands behind his back and handcuffing him. The officer lifted up the attacker, spreadeagled him over the car hood and patted him down. Satisfied, he marched him into the back of the squad car.

Watching the procedure, it dawned on Hank that he had passed a lot of squad cars lately. He was under surveillance. And never realized it.

"We need to fill out a form on this." The police officer had a notebook in his hand.

"I'll fill it out later. You saw it all!" Hank angrily jumped into his car and made a U-turn.

At the hospital, he parked illegally, at the lab entrance. "Where does Blodgett stay when he comes to town?" Hank asked the secretaries.

Two motels were named.

Hank left. Arriving at the first named motel, The Riverview, he asked for Blodgett's room number.

The clerk looked at him strangely. "The police just picked him up."

"How long ago?"

"Five minutes."

Hank thanked the clerk and moved to his car.

The clerk ran to the door. "If you're a friend of his, tell him we don't want his business anymore. We don't like the police coming here like that!"

Hank drove to the police station. Chief Enzer was drinking coffee and staring into space.

"You've got Blodgett."

"Yep."

"I want him."

"Not for a while."

"Why not?"

"Suspicion."

"I was going to make him feel real unhappy." Hank spoke the words slowly.

"Have something to do with the fight you just had?"

"Yep. Why didn't you tell me you were following me everywhere?"

The question was ignored. "We've thrown his hired hand into the holding tank. It may be a few days," said the chief.

"Fill out some papers. A&B Report. Any question in your mind that he and Blodgett are connected? No? None in ours either. Still, we have to be careful—he does work for a large company who might bring in some Fancy-Dan lawyers."

Hank nodded with frustration.

Thirty-seven

Tim quietly looked at him over the desk. Expression-less. His black features seemed to darken with his serious mien.

"We're seeing a lot of each other." Hank spoke quietly.

"Thanks for coming up."

They both sat, reluctant to begin, but knowing it had to be initiated by Tim.

"Doctor...I don't know how to say this but you have become a controversial person. It's difficult to have you around because of all the passions surrounding your presence. Dr. Havermann, our chief of staff, filed a formal complaint against you."

Tim looked down, took a deep breath and let it out slowly. While he did so, Hank wondered what it was like to be a mentally keen administrator, working for numbers of arrogant doctors who demanded, demanded, all day, every day, because of their credentials. He decided he wouldn't like it at all.

"You have a tough job," Hank observed.

Tim smiled ruefully. "I picked the job. Nobody twisted my arm."

Hank nodded. "But people change, situations change, and as a result, job satisfaction changes." Another silence. Tim kept looking down at the papers on his desk. It was all too true.

Hank tried a change. "You're leaving here. Another job in hospital administration?"

"Trying something else. It hasn't been finalized yet, but the trustees have temporarily appointed George Temple. Please keep it confidential."

"Is anything kept confidential in a hospital?"

"Well... I've been asked...told...to request your resignation."

"No."

"I thought you'd say that. Dr. Havermann said he would go before the medical staff and demand a vote on your membership."

"It's not that easy, Tim. You know no one can force a doctor off the medical staff unless there are grounds for incompetence, poor morals, chemical dependency, or the like. And once voted out, the State Medical Board must be notified and their investigators check to see if the medical license should be lifted. Once a person is on the medical staff, bouncing him or her off is asking for an investigation."

"Allegations are that they have three charges against

you and were hoping you would resign."

"Dr. Haims spearheaded the garbage about incompetence. He's gone now and things seemed to have quieted down. The committee refuses to meet and officially lift my probation, even though they have had my replies to their allegations."

"Well, an...alcohol...question..."

"Who told you about that?"

Tim hesitated, then said, "A doctor."

"Schmidt." Hank shook his head sadly.

Tim looked uncomfortable. "I can understand why you two don't get along. But I had no choice but to make him director."

"Not blaming you. In your job, I might have had to do the same thing. You won't believe me if I say I'm not an alcoholic. Anything else?"

"No."

"Good luck, Tim." Hank got up and left, even though Tim acted like he had more to say. It would be helpful to neither of them. The general conversations about other things would be out of place now.

Hank walked downstairs to the laboratory.

The movement to remove him from the staff was what Haims and his cronies had tried to do from the beginning. Haims was dead and gone, yet still the elaborate methods were working to set him up. Why? It didn't make sense.

"Get the flowers?" It was Dr. Sam Sager who fell in step with Hank.

"Yes. The lab appreciates your thoughtfulness. We were just talking about it."

"Just saying thanks, that's all. You guys work so hard for us with little enough acknowledgement! Understand you had to post another murder!" Sam wrinkled his brow.

"Yes. A friend of mine—Cliff Evers."

"Oh? How'd he die?"

"Have to keep it under wraps. The coroner and the chief want it that way.

"Yeah. I suppose you can't say anything. Did I ever tell you about a patient of mine who had a diagnosis of cancer and had six months to live? He insisted I *had* to do something because he *had* to live longer than six months. I told him to go to Salt Lake City, find a Mormon girl, and move to Butte, Montana. He asked me why he should do that—and I told him if he married that Mormon girl and moved to Butte, that six months would seem like a long, long, *long* time!" Sam made his half-swing and moved away, laughing and laughing.

He unlocked the desk drawer and took out the notes from the surgical charts in medical records. Someone was in the room. Hank startled and ducked, ready for anything.

Quiet, academic Alex was there. The man everyone avoided because he enjoyed talking so long. It was the knowledge that they would be tied up so long if they asked a simple question: each question resulted in a lecture with all its ramifications.

"You're getting closer and closer to the murderer." Alex peered at him over his small octagonal glasses.

Hank took a moment to adjust his thinking. "Yes. I'm very close to the person who committed both murders."

Alex looked pleased. "I've heard you use the word 'skull-duggery.' I think it's apt and I know you'll tell me when you're ready. In the meantime, have you thought to check out, in our lab computer, all the diagnoses we make?"

"If there's something wrong, why didn't you just come and tell me?"

"Inherent weakness for wanting to stay clear of controversy. Until it became pure immorality..."

"Don't say it. 'You didn't want to get involved.'"

"Too prosaic. The work I do, I do well. I cover myself by keeping copies of all my diagnoses. Might I suggest you do the same?"

"Too late, but thanks, Alex."

"In simple words then, keep me in mind if you make any major decisions. I know my strengths and weaknesses and I am available."

"What?" Hank started to say.

But it was to a retreating back. He had learned more about Alex in these few days than he had in all the previous years. Alex was amusing. Hank thought of him as self-assigned to an Imperial Duty, descending, pointing out observable injustices and inadequacies, and returning to his lofty throne. Mere mortals could take it from there.

Just the same, Hank felt appreciative and surprised that Alex had considered him important enough to consider as a partner.

But that was all something else. Alex said to check the lab copies of the surgical diagnoses. Hank had gone to the medical records and recopied everything as before. Now he could compare them.

The computer would check out the final tissue diagnoses. Hank punched in his personal password. Only pathologists could review and correct anatomical diagnoses. None that he listed should correlate with the chart. He had performed the work personally and remembered most of the cases he had copied down. He waited for the green glow to appear in the heading—then began with the first name.

The pathological diagnosis in the lab computer matched the diagnosis in the first patient's record on his list. Hank was stunned. He began to feel sick. It couldn't be! They just couldn't match. Only the diagnosis in the chart should have been changed and instead, the copy in the lab had also been changed! There was no error on his part—he remembered the cases he had selected and his diagnoses. But they matched in the computer! Incorrect diagnosis matched incorrect diagnosis!

He continued down the list. One case after another had been altered. Hank's diagnosis of "Normal appendix" was changed to "Acute appendicitis." "Gall bladder" was changed to "Chronic cholecystitis." "Tonsils and adenoids" were changed to "Chronic hypertrophic tonsillitis and adenoiditis."

Even his diagnosis of "Breast tissue, no pertinent histological change" was converted to "Early fibroadenoma, duct ectasia, intraductal epitheliosis and papillomatosis."

All his diagnoses of normal tissues were categorized into disease states. Only pathologists had access to this computer. Someone with medical knowledge. The diagnoses were too exacting. This meant someone with access to their computer had been redoing their diagnoses.

Why hadn't he thought of this previously? It was almost incomprehensible. He had assumed that Haims was the problem since Haims had the most to gain! Is this what Alex was referring to initially?

He went down the hall to his old office. Dr. Schmidt was there. "Schmidt! Who changed the diagnoses on surgical tissues? I haven't checked the autopsy reports, but I wouldn't be surprised if someone hadn't tampered with those as well. Did you do it?"

Hank tried to judge Schmidt's reaction. Genuine surprise and shock was all that he could interpret. "That's awful!" Schmidt exclaimed. "Diagnoses have been changed? We can't allow that! Who would do something like that? Who would dare?"

"Every surgeon would like to write down his own

pathological diagnosis," Hank said. "You know that! All my diagnoses of normal tissue removal have been changed to disease states! No surgeon's capabilities would be under surveillance this way!"

Schmidt said, "How would an outsider get into our lab computer? We're the only ones who have the passwords and we change them every year."

Hank looked grim. "This has now become more than just a game of changing words around—especially with Medicare rules and felony charges. What government attorney wouldn't be delighted to investigate this type of violation. It's page-one newspaper material."

Schmidt turned pale. His hands began to shake and he got up and sat down in his agitation. Groaning, he said, "If it ever got out, it would ruin everyone's reputation—the hospital's as well as ours!" Schmidt appeared as though he were becoming physically ill.

"The hospital and lab will be smashed. Tim Hawkes knows it's something he can't fix, so he's leaving fast." Hank stuck his hands into his lab pockets and shook his head at the thought. "That's not all that'll be smashed. I've asked chemistry to analyze some blood in the forensic case you saw. The smell tipped me off—it was similar to the Haims case. I've a good idea who did it!"

"Is it someone we know?" Schmidt asked.

"Yes. And know very well," said Hank. "I'll have it worked up this afternoon and later tonight, I'll give the information to the authorities."

Schmidt put his shaking hands over his face. "Hank. I know we have had personal differences with each other, but this calls for unity. I got emotional and screwed up the Haims autopsy. I know it now! But this time, let's take it one step at a time. If you agree, first, let's have a meeting...tonight...just us four. We'll find the culprit and proceed from there."

Schmidt looked up at him, his eyes begging. Embarrassed at such emotion and vulnerability, Hank began to weaken.

"Please!" continued Schmidt. "We're professionals. We can't allow anything like this! Think of all the trusting people who work in this laboratory and hospital...who believe in us! It'll ruin everyone. Let's all meet here at seven tonight when things are quiet and stay until we solve it. Say you'll come!"

"Fine," said Hank, slowly and reluctantly. "I'll come."

"They always said you were a true gentleman!" said Schmidt, his eyes brimming with admiration. "They were right. You won't regret this!"

But it *was* a mistake Hank would regret.

Thirty-eight

When he went home for supper, the smell of corned beef and cabbage revived his spirits. He broke the news at dinner. Immediately, Corky's eye's flashed. A dangerous sign.

"Don't do it!" Corky said. "Don't go. I don't trust him."

"I already agreed. How else can we confront whoever did it and find out who is responsible?"

"Cancel going. You didn't do it so you've nothing to gain."

"Perhaps. But I'm almost on to clearing myself and pinpointing the murderer of Haims and Cliff Evers!"

"Obviously one of the pathologists is involved. You

already know that."

"No, that I don't. I'm not even sure Haims's murder is related to this scam. One of the lab personnel could have gotten our passwords and passed it..."

"Why? What would they gain? And how could they know exactly what technical words to use? You said it was smoothly done so any misspelling would be too obvious. It has to be a pathologist. You have a crook in your own department who is being paid off to change the diagnoses and keep an inept surgeon out of trouble," Corky continued, angry.

"Surgeons. There's more than one. Just the same, a clerk could be persuaded to do it by being given the right words to use," said Hank. "You can't definitely finger a pathologist."

"Are you going to the meeting?"

"Yes."

Corky glared at him. "In spite of my telling you to let someone else handle it! You are out of your field of training. Tell the administrator! Tell the president! If you don't trust him, then tell the executive committee! You're not in the real world! You never were! Dad often said..."

Hank put down his fork and sighed.

Corky continued, "Never mind what he said. You're a bull-headed robot! You're in a snake bed and you don't even know it!"

"I promised to go."

"Then why do you tell me about these things and when you've already made up your mind what you're going to do!

"I don't know."

Corky slammed down the dinner plate and stormed out of the room.

He ate the rest of the meal alone. The corned beef and cabbage was usually his favorite and ordinarily he would have lingered over it. Now, it was almost tasteless.

When he had finished, he rinsed the plate and placed it in the dishwasher as a penance effort. The children typically ignored their conversation, being busy in their own affairs, but this time, they were in and out the room continuously, listening and whispering to each other.

Seven o'clock came quickly enough. Corky did not come downstairs. He'd bring her some flowers when he returned.

The lab at night was typically quiet compared to the daytime. Only a few techs were on duty for emergencies. Often they were gone from the lab, drawing blood from patients on various hospital floors, so that the lab appeared abandoned.

The secretary-phlebotomist was away from her desk. She worked alone. In addition to her regular duties, she had to drive the courier car to the airport or Greyhound bus depot and pick up specimens or blood shipped in from Boise.

He went into his office. A note was on his desk. "Postmortem for Dr. Whipple. Stat please!" It was to be performed as soon as possible.

It was strange that he hadn't been notified on his beeper. Perhaps the night secretary had been too busy to notify him—that sometimes happened.

The chart and permit were probably in the morgue. The door was unlocked and the red light was on, which meant a body was on the table in readiness for an autopsy. As he walked in, he saw a form covered with a sheet.

He looked around the room for the chart or for a permit. Unless the permission was valid, an autopsy couldn't be performed.

There was a knock. A voice shouted outside the door, "Doctor! Pathologist! Are you doing an autopsy? The light is on. Can we watch?" Nursing students.

As he turned toward the door to reply, he sensed someone behind him. It lifted itself off the morgue table, clamped one arm around his neck and at the same moment, smothered his face with a cloth containing a mixture of a gaseous chemical which immediately penetrated into his lungs. So much of the chemical was being splashed over his face that it burned into his mouth and caused him to choke. In seconds, everything went black.

Thirty-nine

The shaking of his body aroused him from semiconsciousness. It was cold but as he tried to pull the covers over
him, his hands moved together and hit something that gave
a dull sound. Metal. He opened his eyes to darkness. He
was blind. He feared blindness. That was the worst of all
worlds when his work depended on eyesight.

He began to panic. Something was in his mouth,
preventing breathing. He spit. It wouldn't come out. He
moved his tongue around and around and pushed. The gag
was stuck to the roof of his dry mouth. Finally, the soft
material left his mouth. He could now breathe better.

Concentrating on pushing the stuff from his mouth

somehow cleared his brain. He was aware of his chattering teeth and shaking body even more. His face and mouth burned.

Cramped. He was in something. Cold. A box. A motor was running. A refrigerator. He was in a refrigerator. Only the morgue refrigerator would be this big and long. He tried to move his arms. They wouldn't move. They were tied together. So were his feet. The knees. He could bend his knees.

Claustrophobic fear started to take over. He began to shout. The sound was muffled around his ears and reverberated. He tried to bang on the metal walls. Not loud enough.

Sense! He had to make sense.

The door. Where was the door? Find the door. Door. Find the door. The thought keep repeating itself. Nothing. Smooth walls everywhere. It couldn't be. There had to be a door crack! Something. How stupid! Wrong wall. He was feeling the back of a refrigerator. He rolled over and felt a crack and a lining of soft plastic material. That was it. Push! Nothing. Keep pushing. Still no movement. It was the door, wasn't it? Bend the knees, dummy! Then push!

His mind felt congealed but time was short. He had to tell himself to count. Bend the knees. He felt them come up...shaking. Now tuck them under your chin! Order it. Command it! On three. One. Two. Three! Now! Again! One. Two. Three!

The refrigerator door flew open with a bang. Warm air struck him. Welcome. Warmth never felt so good! He rolled onto the horizonal door. The latches partially bent under his weight as he tumbled to the morgue floor. Thank God the refrigerator was ancient. One of the cost-control measures of the hospital. With better latches he would have been...

He lay there in the dark and saw a small crack of light under the entrance door to the morgue. The refrigerator motor cut into his thoughts with its rumble.

He could see after all! His eyes hurt so badly. But at least he could see! Gratefully, he looked at the crack of light with one eye and then tried the other. Both eyes worked.

A surge of relief covered him and warmed him so that he hopped up to a standing position and moved to the opposite side of the room where he knew the drawer contained the scalpels, large knives, and bone cutters.

Halfway there he realized he had passed the light switch. He could turn on the lights. He hopped back and hit the switch with his shoulder. Light flooded the room like an enveloping; a protecting sun. His hands were tied with the same twine they used to sew up the bodies.

Soft footsteps penetrated the silence outside the door of the morgue. Too soft. The knob was turning quietly. No one entered the morgue without knocking and waiting. This person was not waiting for permission to enter.

The assailant was coming back to finish the job.

He thought of shouting. It wouldn't do any good. The Morgue was located in the lower basement of the hospital. Hank pulled out the drawer. Everything fell on the ground. Quickly, he bent down and tried to pick up the largest-handled knife with his tied hands. It slipped from his grasp and went skittering across the floor as the door quickly opened.

Forty

The figure was covered in a surgical gown, mask and hat. Two deadly eyes pierced the lighted room. One glance at the opened refrigerator door and another to Hank's corner was all that was needed to sum up what had happened. The eyes trained on Hank were merciless.

Fear paralyzed Hank. Flight was impossible. His arms were numb and his legs wouldn't obey. *No*, he thought.

His brain began to convulse as the assailant approached, gravely intent on what he was to do, with a lack of emotion that was unnerving.

"*No!*" Hank heard himself shout—his angry voice was mixed with shattering fear. The commanding voice caused the killer to hesitate a moment. Then, reaching down, he yanked on both of Hank's tied legs. As Hank splattered down to the floor, he felt his head bounce off the side of the drawers and bump on the handles.

A loaded syringe was in the killer's hand. It was held up to the light as air was quickly expressed out of it. Habit. No need for that! A habit by a doctor or nurse. His assailant was trained for helping life. Now it was being used for death. The moment was enough to give Hank a chance to raise himself.

As the killer bent over him, Hank jackknifed his body, bringing his knees to his chin and kicked as hard as he could. He met air and felt wretched and foolish.

The killer had skipped away. Now, he rapidly approached.

Instantly, Hank repeated the jackknife, this time twisting his direction. The killer had misjudged how fast Hank could recoup and tried to dodge again, only to receive the kick to his head, both of Hank's feet forming a V underneath the chin. The syringe spun out of his hand but the blow was partly a spent force. The killer stumbled and tried to regain his balance, only to overbalance, stagger, then slip on the syringe. His forehead crashed against the sharp edge of the morgue table. The sound was a sickening, loud crack.

It happened so quickly. The killer's body collapsed after bouncing and rolling. The surgical cap fell to the floor and the mask hung down, twisted around his neck. He felt the mixture of emotions draining his strength when he saw who the killer was.

His throat hurt so badly! Get out of here. Hurry!

He couldn't move until the ropes were cut on his wrists and legs. It seemed to take forever for the knife to cut through morgue twine.

Hank opened the door, gratefully breathing in the air.

Looking back, he found he couldn't leave without checking the body for vital signs. Habit. Like expressing air from a syringe before injecting. There were no vitals.

Sam Sager was dead.

Forty-one

Voices were coming down the hall. Corky, Chief Enzer and Monty appeared.

"What...you...doing here?" asked Hank, half-dazed.

"Your wife brought us."

"Why?" The word came out as a croak.

"You didn't answer your page and weren't in the building, so she got worried." Aftershock. He became aware of the burning pain.

Hank went back into the morgue to a large sink and put his head under the running water. It felt good. The pain began to ease. He filled his mouth with water and spit. It didn't matter what it looked like. He stuck both arms under the welcome fluid.

"Always bathe in chemicals?" That was Monty. Quiet. Questioning.

Bathe? Thanks, Monty. He had forgotten the shower next to the morgue.

The refrigerator door was still open.

Sam Sager lay quietly stretched out on the floor. A pool of blood was spreading out under him and moving to the floor drain.

"Oh!" said Corky after one glance and left the room quickly.

In a daze, water dripping down his face and onto his clothes, Hank tried to whisper what had happened. Only a few words came out.

The chief grunted and made a quick phone call. Within moments, a police team was present.

He recognized them all. He had taught autopsy procedure to most of them when they were rookies. The picture-taking began and the fingerprint boys moved in.

"Wish you hadn't washed, Doc. Might have picked up an interesting print or two. Now it's just your word against his."

"Couldn't...help it," rasped Hank, apologetically.

They grinned at him. Funny. He had missed the gallows humor. He began to laugh, but coughed instead.

Corky was back but carefully avoided looking downward. She explained, "When Dr. Schmidt called a meeting for seven o'clock tonight, I told Hank not to go. He insisted. When no one had seen any of the pathologists here, I called you." Corky first glared at Hank fiercely and then looked at him sympathetically.

"What kind of meeting?" asked Monty.

"Long story," gasped Hank.

"We've got plenty of time."

"I'll...write it," Hank whispered tiredly. Waves of nausea were beginning to spread over him. He couldn't get sick here. He wouldn't. He wrote as quickly as he could.

"Typical doctor's handwriting," grunted the chief, trying to read the scribble. "Why didn't he simply bash you on the head or garrote you?"

Hank wrote.

"So you were lucky! If the nurses hadn't knocked on the door and interrupted him—he had just enough time to throw you into the refrigerator and skip out the back door as the nurses came in the front. Then he had to return to finish the job."

Hank smiled weakly.

"This ties up the loose ends." The chief looked to Monty for agreement, but Monty's voice could be heard outside talking to the laboratory night crew.

Just like Monty, thought Hank, disbelieving what I've said until he has checked out everything and everyone and has their signatures on their statements.

The thought was bittersweet. Bitter because they still didn't quite believe him, and yet he knew Monty was doing a thorough job—probably just as Hank would have done in reversed circumstances.

Corky drove him home and he looked forward to a rest. His throat was raw and hurt. Monty was at his home within fifteen minutes of his own arrival.

Insistent but patient, Monty wrote down what Hank tried to indicate with single words and nods of the head. After reading the sequence of events as he had dictated, Hank signed the notes where Monty indicated.

Forty-two

The next two days he stayed home. Flowers and good wishes arrived from all directions. The newspapers were full of the details. He read them with mental detachment—as though it had all happened to someone else. He expected the newspaper reporters and photographers would be persistent and they were.

The children were pressed into service to bring in the mail from the highway postbox. They were cautioned not to say anything—an impossible task for a child.

Corky tried to be patient with the phone inquiries but finally gave up, took the phone off the cradle, detached the doorbell and locked the doors.

Only Alex was admitted into the house and he carried messages of concern from the laboratorians, hospital staff and the administrator.

"I asked you before if it was worth it," said Alex after accepting a glass of beer. "Well?"

"No. It wasn't worth it!" exclaimed Corky before Hank could reply. "It was silly and stupid!"

"No. It wasn't worth it...but I had to clear myself," said Hank slowly. "I just couldn't let them blame me for Haims's murder."

"The police would have solved it! That's their full-time job, isn't it?" Corky glared at Hank.

"Yes, eventually, I suppose, but..." Hank shrugged.

Alex interrupted. "I'm sorry. Would you summarize what it was all about?"

"Sam Sager killed Haims. You know that," said Hank.

"But why?"

"My guess: Sager was tired of being needled and subjected to Haims's ridicule. When Haims had the quality assurance committee officially reprimand him, it was too much."

"There has to be more to it than that."

"Yes. Haims told me the *exact* percentage of work he brought into the hospital. This, to me at least, meant he wanted more. Sam was a popular physician with the next largest patient census. Since Haims couldn't directly sabotage him, he used the fact that no surgeon is going to make a perfect judgment call each time—especially under pressure. Haims seized on a few unfortunate outcomes that Sager worked on and blew these up out of proportion."

"Ignoring his own," interjected Alex.

"Right. Ignoring any of his own cases that had the same or worse outcome. Hindsight being 100 percent accurate, as chairman, he could review any surgical chart and finger whomever he wanted."

"...and have his bullies go after them."

"Yes."

"What about Cliff? How did that cowboy get into it?"

"Cliff tracked Haims and for weeks, he sat outside Haims's home in a car—staring at the house—until Haims filed a complaint with the police."

"Unsettled?"

"He had reason...his marriage, for one thing...Haims's surgery. I take it he saw Sam Sager visit Haims."

"But the murders were different, weren't they?" asked Corky. "I thought killers repeated themselves...their methods, I mean."

Alex smiled. "Yes, they do. There were similarities—both were bashed in the head from behind and both had lethal injections—insecticide, no less—in the same locations. Am I correct?"

"Yes. You snuck a look at the post-mortem findings," said Hank. "It was one of the common organic phosphates."

"You never told me where the injections were," said Corky, looking blank.

Hank was silent, so Alex replied, "Surgeons, in emergencies, don't bother with veins and arteries in the limbs, Corky. Murdering someone might be termed a sort of emergency procedure, perhaps."

"But where then?"

Alex brought up his thumb and stabbed the left front of his chest, then made a gasping sound and clutched his heart.

"Oh! How awful!" she exclaimed. "I'm sorry I asked. But the police had to know what you knew! Why didn't the police suspect Dr. Sager?"

"Reasonable alibi. He made sure he was performing

surgery at the time with plenty of witnesses attesting to it. Forgotten is the time-lapse between cases, in which the room has to be cleaned, new packages of surgical instruments brought in—not to speak of the time required to place the patient under anesthesia. Sam Sager could say he was in surgery, run out, do his deeds and return."

"That leaves Stan Schmidt. He has simply disappeared. You understand his role in all of this?" asked Alex.

Hank sighed. "I suspect his payoff was receiving my job. He tipped off Sam Sager that I knew who the killer was. Schmidt was in it very deeply. I figure Schmidt had two different discs in the computer—one for the correct diagnoses and the other for the ones he altered. He could switch back and forth as needed—a consultant would receive the original and correct diagnosis."

"How did you figure it was Sam Sager?" asked Alex.

"Large, bulky body described by a student nurse. Coat with a fur collar. But more so, when I watched Sam's mannerism in swinging. It was like he was bashing something."

Alex shook his head sadly. "Sam Sager was such an accomplished raconteur. It's hard to say some of us will miss a killer. By the way, your job—or former job—is now open again, since Dr. Schmidt cannot be located. Interested?"

Hank blocked the question. "How about the administrator? What's happening with him?" he asked.

"Tim left for job in a small town in Wisconsin. George is maintaining the status quo until a replacement is found."

"George can't handle the shrapnel that's to come."

"He'll have to bear it because the hospital is under investigation."

"What'll they find?"

"Massive confusion. Everything in a flux. The nuns are

most unhappy about the direction of the hospital. For one thing, you caught their attention with your avalanche of memos about the problems with the diagnostics—they're not going to be so adamant about all the contracts being bid out of Minnesota."

"Like central government," smiled Hank ruefully.

"With similar results," offered Alex.

Forty-three

"Welcome back!" said Ruth, the ever-loyal tech. Three days were all. He was back at St. Mary's in Schmidt's old office.

Hank looked up to reply and saw that the outside corridor behind her was filled with laboratorians. The chief tech was grinning and waving. Alex stood silently behind them.

"Well...it's quite a welcome! Thank you," Hank stuttered, hoping he sounded appreciative enough through his embarrassment.

"Come with us!" commanded Carol.

He followed them to the break room, which they had

decorated with signs of "Welcome" and "Our Hero!" Pastries and fresh coffee filled the large table. It was heartwarming and fun.

Just the same, some important personal decisions had to be made—continuing on at St. Mary's was different now. The first day back, he was the focal point of interest in the surgical lounge. As usual, the sentences were hurried and the words staccato—patients' needs came first.

"Absolutely amazing. Two surgeons are dead. Both are the top guns in the hospital."

"Fighting is one thing; actual murder..Incomprehensible!"

Then the macabre humor: "Whipple—it's too hot in here, do you know a quick way a guy can cool off? Do you have a cold slot in the lab?"

Disbelief, belief, some admiration, some not—all in all, the same questions were answered and reanswered.

Both surgeons left a large gap that had to be filled right away. A search team was formed to interest two general surgeons to practice at Red Wolf.

Life went on and the work would continue, thought Hank. How long before they completely forgot the incident?

Blodgett was left high and dry by his company when their preliminary investigations revealed that he hired thugs to enforce his sales territory.

Mother Superior contacted him and asked him to be acting director and order whatever supplies he needed from his own selected sources, temporarily.

A quick conference with the supervisors enabled them to agree on which firms to use. All Hempter reagents were returned.

"It's a much happier place here now," volunteered Meagan. The relaxed chatter confirmed the increase in morale.

Hank felt satisfied, except the peeling skin over his face and the sloughing which of pieces of gunk from his throat every time he coughed, made him uncomfortable.

An angry Ed Wilkins stared at him. "Here are your bone marrows and a few cases requiring more study," said Wilkins, disgruntled. "I just didn't have time to do your work and mine, too!"

Few cases? "You even left the Pap smears," Hank observed. "Three days?"

"I just can't do it all! It's just too much!"

Hank groaned and shook his head. He coughed and felt something burn deep down in his chest and visualized the dead mucosal lining peeling from the bronchi. Too much learning maketh a fearful man. Seeing things through a microscope all the time wasn't the most calming of experiences when it involved yourself.

Ed Wilkins was still standing there when he looked up. "I might as well tell you that it's irresponsible calling in at the last minute and saying you're not coming into work. It's simply unacceptable!" Ed sputtered as he talked. "I'm going to bring this up at the next meeting—"

"Ed," cut in Hank. "Did you hear about Dr. Sager going bonkers and trying to kill me?"

"Yes." Worry lines appeared on Wilkins's face. "Tell me. What was it all about?" The switch from antagonism to oozing warmth and companionship was made without a trace of embarrassment. One moment outraged and the next moment, solicitous.

"Bug off, Ed," said Hank quietly. "You're too much."

"If you say so," Ed said. He paused, thought a moment and his face changed. He remembered Hank was the acting boss.

"Hank," whimpered Ed. "I'm sorry about not getting more done, but Schmidt quit the hospital without notice.

No one knows where he went. I've been doing his work, too."

"Goodbye, Ed." How could Ed shrug off that he was almost killed?

"I mean, it's not my fault. Really. I'm completely scheduled-out with all kinds of responsibilities!"

"Ed."

"Yes."

"Beat it. Now!"

"God! You can sure turn nasty." Ed left in a swirl of righteous indignation that stayed in the room minutes after he left. An unpleasant aura. Some people did that to every room they were in. Haims. Spans. Schmidt. Wouldn't it be a delight to work with colleagues you had selected and not the ones who had been selected for you?

He began to work as rapidly as possible, knowing the clinicians would be calling for their diagnoses, disgruntled at the delay. Tissue reports were expected to be out the next day. Today was the fourth day. Sure enough. The secretary was at the door.

"Dr. Mullins wants to know the diagnosis on the thyroid he took out a week ago. The patient is in his office now."

Hank sighed. Predictable Mullins. Four days ago was a week to him. Worse yet, Mullins actually believed it was a full seven days. "I'll call him back in a few minutes—just as soon as I read it."

"He sounded angry." The secretary was upset. She was new at handling doctors. She'd learn.

"Just tell him I'll call him back within fifteen minutes."

Most surgeon-doctors sounded angry when a diagnosis was delayed. Hank picked up the slide and groaned. Papillary carcinoma. Cancer. Hopefully focal. Was it?

He followed the capsule—the outside rim—of the

gland and groaned again. The capsule was invaded in several places. Was a frozen section done? He checked. Yes. Ed had deferred the diagnosis. The cancer was in the frozen section slide. They'd have to have a departmental meeting about this and have Ed explain.

Only five minutes had elapsed when Hank picked up the phone and anticipated the barrage of questions—including why the cancer wasn't found at frozen section. He could only reply, "I don't know." The conversation with Dr. Mullins ended amicably.

Telling a patient she had cancer was the hard part. At times like this, the easy part was looking through the microscope. Hank put the phone down with a sigh.

The room still had a singular foul aura which spoke of Ed Wilkins and Schmidt. Odious black vapors seemed to permeate the entire room. Almost unbearable.

"Staying here or leaving? Any decisions, Master? Speak! I beg of thee!" Alex walked in and sat down heavily in a chair.

Hank laughed. Alex had picked a vulnerable time.

"Leaving."

"Finally! At long last!" exclaimed Alex. "You are known for being persistent but nice, and unreasonable but nice. I wondered when the unreasonable would emerge! The nice was beginning to get ridiculous...where are we going?"

"Across from the hospital," said Hank, surprised at the certainty in his voice. "Hold on. Are you sure about the we?"

"What are we going to name the laboratory?" asked Alex, smiling broadly at the ceiling.

"Umm...The Pathologist's Laboratory," said Hank.

"Too mundane. Vision is what is needed, Whipple! Luckily, you now have a partner who is not so circumscribed in his thinking! Let's call it, Pathologists' National

Diagnostic Laboratories, Inc. The word *national* has a nice ring to it."

"How about shortening it to Pathologists' National Laboratories?" asked Hank.

"'Incorporated' is at the end. We're going big time, Whipple. Provincialism be damned! What are your plans— I know you have them!" Alex smacked his hands together.

"How did you know?" asked Hank, surprised.

"Rick—the banker. Or should I say, the hospital's banker."

"That's right—he refused me the loan." The thought still rankled. "The Troy Bank was very solicitous. My friend George Maisner has been ready to go on the building part."

"Smart people at Troy! What do we have for corporate philosophy? Let's come to an agreement on this first." Alex's eyes narrowed.

"Alex, you're full of surprises. I wasn't aware you cared about anything but academic work!"

"A phase. Now...on to practicing independently, as true physician-pathologists, instead of hired hands in a hospital! Answer the question, please!"

"Well...very low prices and accurate, rapid turnaround times on analyses...that is, same-day reports," said Hank. "Also an extensive courier system with part-time techs...until volume expands."

"Sending out sales reps bother you as unethical... unprofessional?" inquired Alex. "How about advertising? Competing with other labs?"

"All necessary."

"Agreed! Let's shake on it." Alex offered both hands.

ABOUT THE AUTHOR

Harry Chinchinian lives on a high broad hill above the Snake River in Washington in more or less harmony with an amused wife, a dozen perpetually hungry horses, and two devoted Irish Wolfhounds.

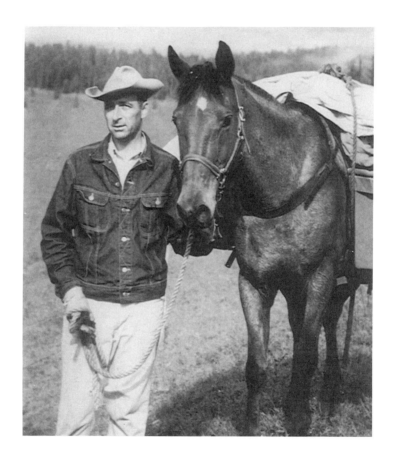

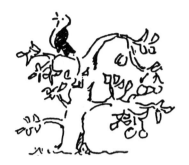

Plum Tree Press
531 Silcott Road Clarkston, WA 99403
Order Form

Pathologist In Peril _____ x 8.95 = _____
Immigrant Son (Soft cover) _____ x 7.95 = _____
Immigrant Son (Hard cover) _____ x 18.95 = _____
                    Postage and Handling _____ =   2.00
                                         Total _____

_____Check enclosed

_____VISA   Account #_____
_____MC   Exp. Date_____

                   Signature_____

Name _____
Address _____
City/State _____Zip_____
Phone (   )_____

**Plum Tree Press   531 Silcott Road
                         Clarkston, WA 99403
                         1-800-799-8829**